FOREST BATHING IN THE ADIRONDACKS

A Guide for
House or Forest

HOLLY CHORBA

Copyright © 2025 by Holly Chorba

All rights reserved.

No portion of this book may be reproduced in any form without written permission from the publisher or author and photographer except as permitted by U.S. copyright law.

ISBN: 979-8-9855013-2-2

ISBN: 979-8-9855013-1-5

The Peace of the Wild Things
by
Wendell Berry

"When despair for the world grows in me, and I wake
in the night at the least sound in fear of what my life and my
children's lives may be,

I go and lie down where the wood drake rests in his
beauty on the water, and the great heron feeds.

I come into the peace of wild things who do not tax
their lives with the forethought of grief.

I come into the presence of still water. And I feel
above me the day-blind stars waiting with their light.

For a time, I rest in the grace of the world, and am free."

from
The Peace of the Wild Things and Other Poems (Penguin, 2018)

PREFACE

Our natural areas, especially our forests, are quickly disappearing. Our lifestyles more and more frequently surround us with traffic, noise, artificial lights, pollution, buildings, cement, and crowds of people we do not know.

Joni Mitchell put it succinctly in her song "Big Yellow Taxi" (1970). "You don't know what you've got till it's gone…They've paved paradise and put up a parking lot." Even back as far as 1873, Henry David Thoreau stated, "In wilderness is the preservation of the world." Our natural world needs us for its preservation!

The Environmental Defense Fund (EDF) Impact 2023 report, "Finding Solutions in Nature," stated, "Nature plays a crucial role in solving the climate crisis by storing carbon in soils, trees, and the deep ocean. Protecting forests offers the single largest natural climate solution. But our science shows that the risk to forests is growing, in part due to climate change itself. "We recognize the value in that "EDF is laser-focused in accelerating investments in forest protection worldwide."

Mankind sees the problem and knows that it is us. We resort to the bath or similar quiet, comforting experiences to relax away from all that hubbub, or we seek vacation in a less busy area such as New York State's Adirondack region. A new kind of bath, in the forest, offers a personal restorative experience that can connect us with long advocated Nature. First developed in Japan as an antidote to extreme urbanization, "Forest Bathing" is now practiced worldwide.

ACKNOWLEDGMENTS

Forest Bathing and the Adirondacks are each dear to my heart! They make me and so many others happy!

This book is also written to increase your happiness too. It serves as an introduction to Forest Bathing and to the Adirondacks. May you also appreciate them. I sincerely believe that appreciation is the very key to happiness!

I dedicate this volume to those responsible for my knowledge, love, and enjoyment of the Adirondacks, most especially to my late husband Ronald Chorba, who twice back-packed the Northville-Placid Trail in its entirety with me, and took me on many spectacular hikes, beautiful paddling and waterfall adventures, and memorable canoe/camping trips with friends and family. Also, I dedicate it to my premier paddling buddy, Carolyn Kaczka, who was the inspiration for my increased exploration and enjoyment of so many aspects of the Park, including its rivers and lakes, less famous mountains, its art, architecture, history, literature, museums, and even its culinary delights.

The connection and appreciation of the Adirondack Woods ' healing power has been made more accessible to even the most reticent urbanite with the introduction of the practice of Forest Bathing.

Practitioners Helene Gibbons and Suzanne Weirich introduced me to Forest Bathing. Since then, I have had the privilege of participating with others in such guided walking/sensory experiences led by Debra Mitchell and Sarah Pickard. Sally Hartman, Greg Smith, and Cynthia Grover accompanied me on several adventures. Sarah and her teenage friend Lariah Anne served as models for my photography.

Others, more distantly related, have been major influences on my appreciation. I was privileged to meet and converse with

Clarence Petty, former forest ranger, naturalist, and advocate of the Adirondack Park. The late Peter Hornbeck, who built many ADK canoes and painted lovely ADK scenes, was largely responsible for the practicalities of my solo paddling. Sandra Hildreth, ADK landscape painter, Carl Heilman, ADK photographer, and Ed Katz, Naturalist, all enhanced my appreciation of ADK Park. Historic figures also figured importantly: tuberculosis researchers including E.L. Trudeau; Adirondack guide and hotelier Paul Smith; the Hermit Noah Rondeau; and photographer and writer Seneca Ray Stoddard. Authors, listed in the Citations, have informed me over the years of what a tremendous resource we have in New York State's Adirondacks.

Largely through Carolyn Kaczka I became familiar with the author Martha Reben (The Healing Woods, 1952). Ms. Reben was a tuberculosis patient at Saranac Lake. Reflecting on her recovery, confirmed after 10 summers spent at a primitive camp on Weller Pond, she wrote:

"Now that I was strong enough to walk…to wander in the woods… there was an endless fascination coming from the dim, almost cathedral solemnity of the pine and hemlock into the sunny…gay openness of birch and beech and maple woods. From there…into the balsam swamp with a brook, and a lush patch of ferns…(pushing) my way noisily through dry and crackling twigs…into woods almost open. The wilderness did more than heal my lungs, however… with its tranquility, it bestowed upon me …a sense of freshness and wonder which life in natural surroundings daily brings and a joy in the freedom, beauty, and peace that exist in a world apart from human beings."

Of course, Carolyn and I pilgrimaged by canoe to that Weller Pond camp!

Ashley Cunningham, Sally Hartman and Lariah Anne, Cynthia Grover, Greg Smith, Sandra Hildreth, Donna Andre, Beth Mosher, and Francoise Goodrow have all joined me in several more adventures in the Adirondack Park.

Friends and former English teachers Valerie Dunning and Joyce Monroe have served as editors.

My team at the nativepublishers.com, especially have been instrumental in formatting, producing, and marketing this book.

Read further for an explanation of what "Forest Bathing" is, sample an introductory Forest Bath, and read how the vast northeastern Adirondack Forest has a long history, continuing to the present day, of being a "healing wood."

TABLE OF CONTENTS

PART I. FOREST BATHING 1

PART II. YOUR FOREST BATH 6

PART III: THE ADIRONDACKS 54

PART IV: CITATIONS AND RESOURCES 63

PART I. FOREST BATHING

"Forest Bathing"... the very term conjures up visions of wood nymphs shedding their gossamer gowns and entering limpid vernal pools surrounded by lacy ferns, accompanied by the melodic song of birds and adorned with flitting pastel butterflies. I was enchanted the first time I heard the term, *Forest Bathing,* yet I have learned it is not that vision at all. Still, I have remained enchanted with Forest Bathing for the years that have followed.

I have learned what Forest Bathing is not. Forest Bathing is NOT a fantasy minuet of wood nymphs, nor is it bird watchers seeking a unique species, botanists looking to discover an unknown herb, or hikers bagging a peak in record time. It is not a form of exercise, nor is it competitive, nor is it designed for the professional naturalist seeking to identify each species.

Forest Bathing is focused immersion in nature using the senses to draw attention to the present moment. A Forest Bath is a lot like any bath. It cleanses you. It takes away grime - in this case, the grime of whatever is worrying you, stressing you, or causing you pain. It cleanses thoughts by focusing on observations of what's happening in the forest in the present moment. It is a self-care strategy, a method to improve health and reconnect with the natural world. It can decrease the level of the stress hormone cortisol as phytoncides released by trees impact the human body. It has been shown to improve heart rate variability and blood pressure, decrease anxiety and depression, and boost the immune system, which fights off infection and cancer. ("A Dose of Nature" Krempa, 2022; Clifford, 2018)

The practice of Forest Bathing follows guidelines inspired by the Japanese practice of shinrin-yoku. The term was coined in Japan in 1982 by Tomohyde Akiyama, then director of the Japanese Forestry Agency. It was formalized in the United States by M. Amos Clifford in 2012 when he founded the Association of Nature and

Forest Therapy Guides and Programs (ANFT). Today, the practice of Forest Bathing has grown internationally. It generally follows Clifford's design, the design that still enchants me and that I've adapted for my personal use. (Clifford, 2018).

Certified Guides in America can be found through the website https:www.anft.earth/guides. Certified Guides Helene Gibbons and Suzanne Weirich of Adirondack Riverwalking, Saranac Lake, NY, provided my first formal and very alluring Forest Bathing experience. I was awarded that Forest Bathing experience in 2016 for a winning photographic entry in Paul Smith's Visitor Interpretive Center's "Life on the Lakes" juried art show. Thus, from the start, I linked my love of photography to the practice of Forest Bathing. I took part in a formal Helene Gibbons' Forest Bathing (shirin-yoku) group of six adults. That experience and her website (adirondackriverwalking.com) were great introductions to the subject.

Since that day, I have taken part in other such therapeutic woodland walks, researched Forest Bathing, and written and photographed "A Forest Fungi Bath" (Chorba 2017), which introduces those who love the artistry and delicacy of mushrooms to the many colorful types that bedeck the northeastern forests, to the focal vocabulary of mycology, and to the practice of Forest Bathing. Forest Bathing itself has a much wider appeal.

A "Forest Therapy Walk" in November of 2023 guided by Debra Mitchell offered a similar nature immersion experience, found through the Adirondack Mountain Club, Laurentian Chapter. My third official experience was a talk and walk given by ANFT Certified Guide, Sarah Pickard of Lazy River Forest Therapy at lazyriverplayground.com.

Each encounter was very satisfying; each encounter left me eager for another and eager to share the practice of Forest Bathing with you.

Forest Bathers select a site for their *"Bath"* and do well to be appropriately clothed and otherwise prepared. Research where to go and what will make you comfortable and safe. Get dressed for the area and weather (hiking boots? long sleeves? umbrella?). Take what you need (this book? map? insect repellent? cell phone? notepad? drinking water? etc.) to the *"Threshold"* or point where you enter the natural area. Make ready what you will want to have with you as you conclude your experience, perhaps an innocuous "wild" tea such as Chaga or Reishi and a snack such as nuts, berries, or an apple.

Those not yet familiar with *Forest Bathing*, and those unfamiliar with the natural area to be visited can especially benefit from a certified guide and a group of 6 or fewer like-minded fellow participants. This book provides a vicarious introduction. I suggest you also explore options available to you that connect you with an ANFT Guide.

Guides seek to shepherd participants such that observations and perceptions are focused, rumination on negative thoughts is avoided, distractions are eliminated, and the experience of each person is enhanced by the group. The *"Bathers"* engage in a series of deliberate sensory *"invitations"* or suggestions of where to direct their attention. Each person participates to a self-determined degree. The goal is to commune with nature, share what each participant wishes to do in an orderly fashion, and emerge relaxed, refreshed, and enlivened. What each person notices is expanded and enhanced through periodically sharing with others whatever strikes them as notable.

The Guide and the group begin at a select location, at best, a natural one with few distractions from traffic noise, outsiders, human habitation, and distant voices. An area with trees and a water feature such as a bog, swamp, stream, or pond is ideal. The Guide issues *"invitations"* or suggestions to the participants to notice specific aspects of their surroundings using each sense in turn.

Periodically, he or she may pass a *"speaking piece,"* a selected stone or branch, to indicate when a bather may seize the opportunity to speak to the group about his perceptions. Generally, all members of the group are silent between i*nvitations* until passed the *speaking piece*, and each one is passed the *speaking piece* in turn. This limited conversation and banning of the use of technology during the practice facilitates the goal of being one with nature in a relaxed, meditative way. Participants are encouraged to take in what the forest has to give as well as to give thanks back to the forest. The experience is often concluded with a conversation and a wild tea ceremony shared among all participants to summarize and share their thoughts on the *Forest Bathing* experience.

You can begin sampling this type of nature immersion by yourself in a city park, garden, backyard, or quiet room in your house using this book as a substitute for actually being in the forest. Immerse yourself in a vicarious *Forest Bath* in the following pages. Read the *invitations* and contemplate the photographs and poems from my previous Adirondack Forest Bathing experiences, or use the *invitations* to guide you in your own natural setting. You may choose to share your perceptions with a partner, or can mimic sharing by verbalizing your observations, perhaps jotting them down in a notebook and reading some of my earlier B*ath* perceptions in the form of poetry. Such sharing can illuminate what you sense as you contemplate nature.

My photographs are of the Adirondack woodlands, the largest natural area of temperate deciduous forest in the United States. It has an abundance of locations suitable for Forest Bathing. The people photographed include my teenage friend Lariah Anne, Forester Ed Kanze, and certified ANFT Guide, Sarah Pickard.

I became enthralled with the Adirondacks as a six year old when my parents brought me to the area on a camping trip. I have happily lived just beyond the northern border of its six million acre Adirondack Park for more than half a century. Now, enhanced by the practice of *Forest Bathing,* it has become even more of my safe haven, a restorative and meditative retreat from the cares and stresses that can overcome anyone. Please accept this invitation to enjoy your own Forest Bathing experience.

PLEASE NOTE:

Consult guidebooks if you are venturing far afield.

Learn what to avoid and how to protect yourself from potential risks such as from any mosquitos, ticks, poison ivy, venomous reptiles, etc.

Employ a guide in the territory you are unfamiliar with.

Be safe and notify someone of your travels.

Gather your support, such as a map and compass, drinking water, tea, repellent, and a hat.

If you are not used to blocking out thoughts and concentrating only on sensations and observations, you can practice awakening your senses through the many techniques described in <u>Life in Five Senses</u> by Gretchen Ruben (Penguin Random House 2023. ISBN 9780593442746).

Be guided from your coffee table or from your chosen spot in the field.

PART II. YOUR FOREST BATH

You are invited to come bathe with me,
to leave all cares behind, to be present, to just be.
Listen, smell, taste, touch, look.
Behold with your heart!
Give thanks to the forest. Give thanks!
You are one, not apart!

Let's proceed together using the invitations that follow.

Approach your "Threshold," which is your selected spot to enter into your connection with nature. Your Threshold may be the start of a woodland trail, or a comfortable place to sit with this book.

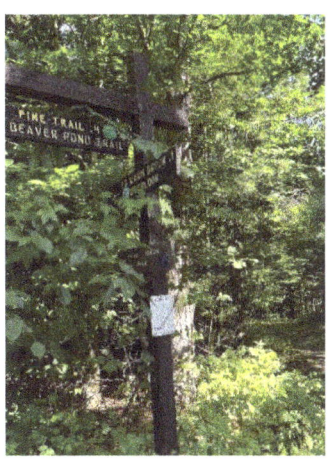
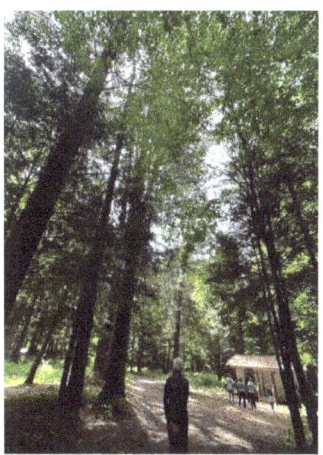
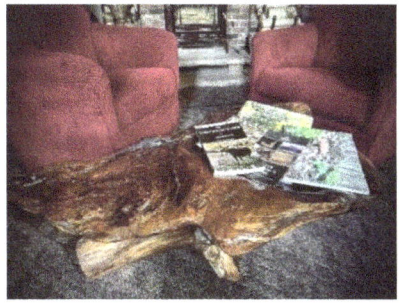

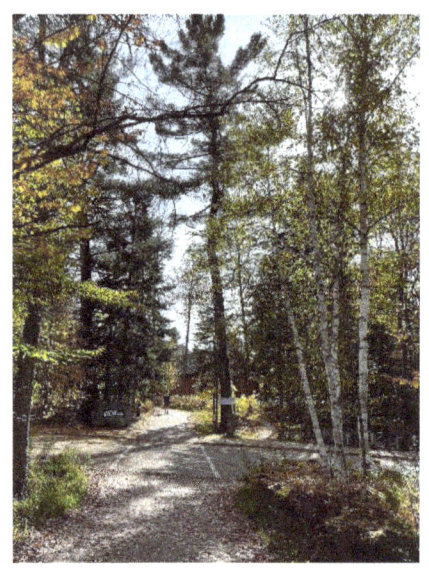
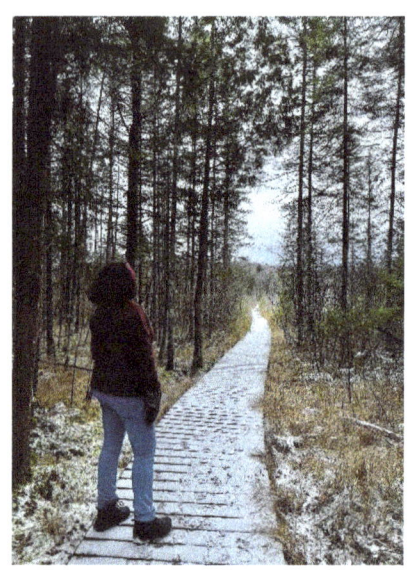
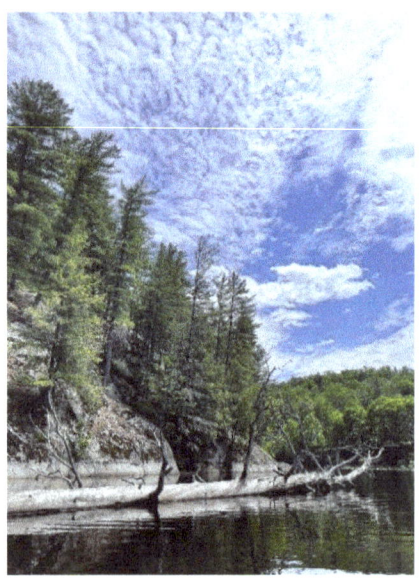
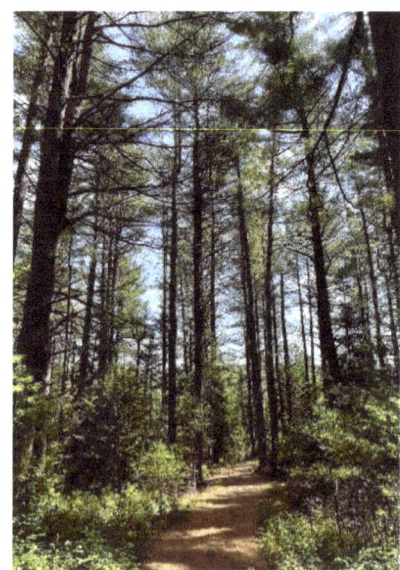

Pause for 15 minutes or so and become aware of intruding thoughts, worries, or pressures to get things done. Shed those distractions like worn clothes.

Bring your attention back to the here and now whenever thoughts of past problems or future worries intrude. Be aware that thoughts are not reality; they are not happening now. They are only in your brain and can be dealt with later. You can exhume them at will after your *Bath*.

Leave your thoughts buried or give them to the clouds or water to carry while you are in your Bath. They will be there when you are finished; no need to carry them with you.

Now perceive the NOW…be mindful only of the present moment.

Focus on the forest.

Now perceive the NOW…be mindful only of the present moment.

Focus on the forest.

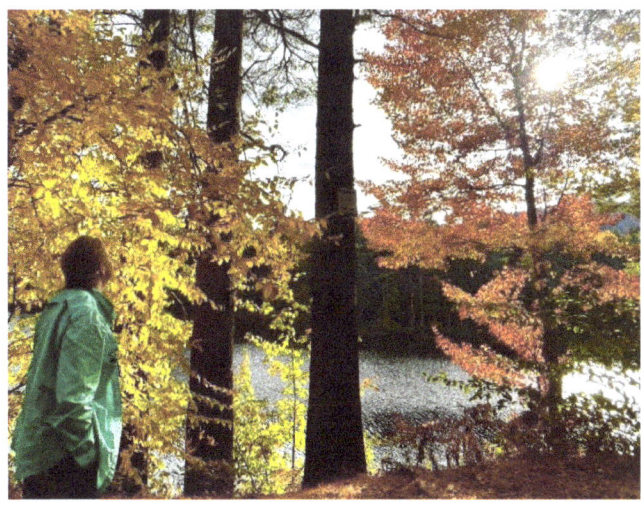

Stand at the threshold of this experience. Get comfortable.
Anticipate being part of the forest for a carefree, relaxed time.
Accept this invitation to BE; be aware of your body.
Feel your position in this space.

Use your proprioception to sense the position of your body in space and its interface with the environment.

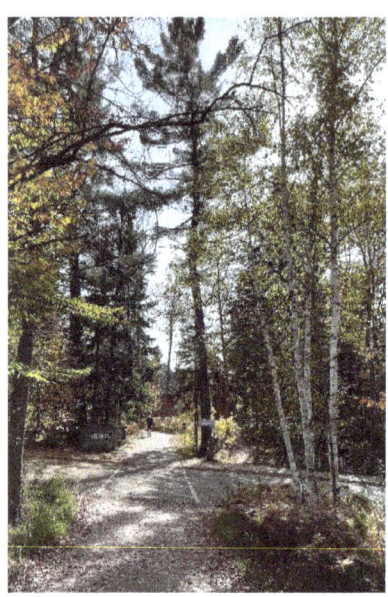
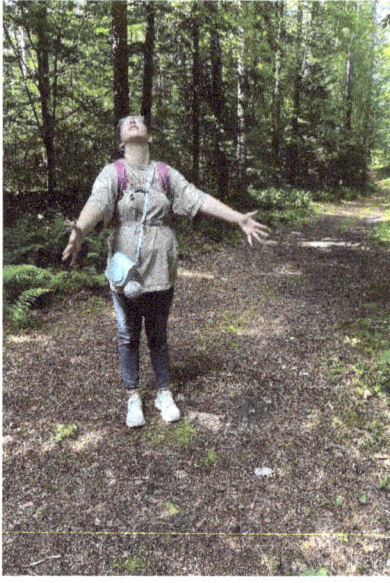

Feel the floor or ground touching your feet. Do you notice pressure? A soft or hard underlayment? Cushion of moss or carpet?

Gently close your eyes and feel the air on your face; feel the position of your knees and legs.

Move gently, letting kinesthesia inform you of your motions. Move your arms and hands gently…up, down…forward, back.

Maintain balance as you bend your knees, shrug your shoulders, and twist your torso.

Open your eyes and turn to face each direction.
Breathe slowly and deeply, in…out…repeat several times.
Feel the air enter and leave your nasal passages and lungs.
Notice how your breath feels coming in…flowing out.
Let the air around you blend with your body.

Your entire body senses its surroundings…awkward, comfortable, warm, cool, free, restricted.

Your body may react to the immediate surroundings by communicating with your brain, resulting in eager enjoyment or boredom or curiosity or enthusiasm.

Shut your eyes and sense your position in space.
Bring your responses back to simple perceptions.
Become aware of what your body is feeling now.

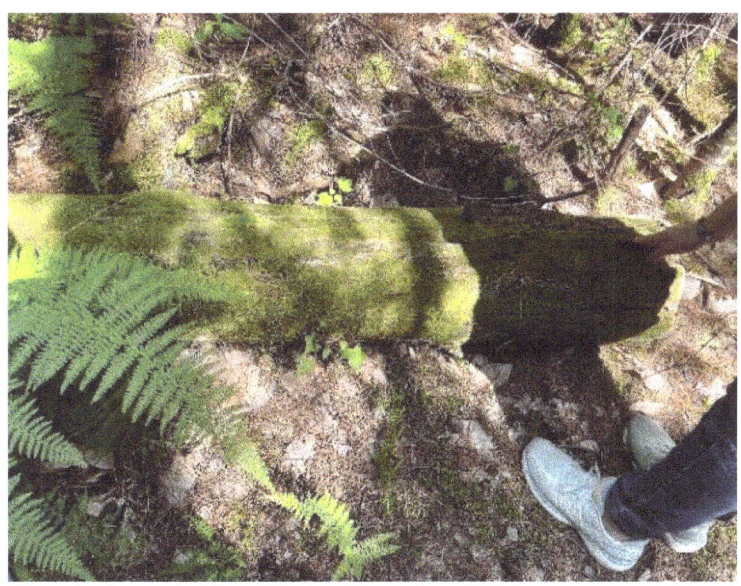

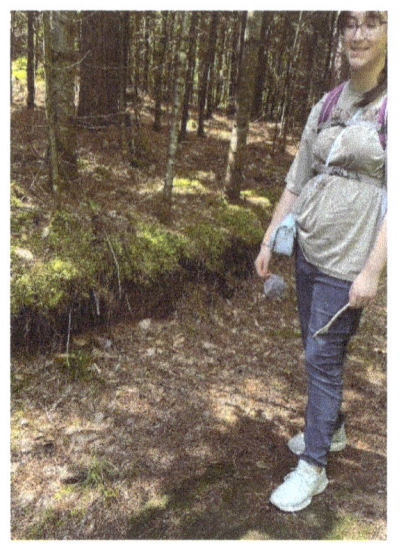
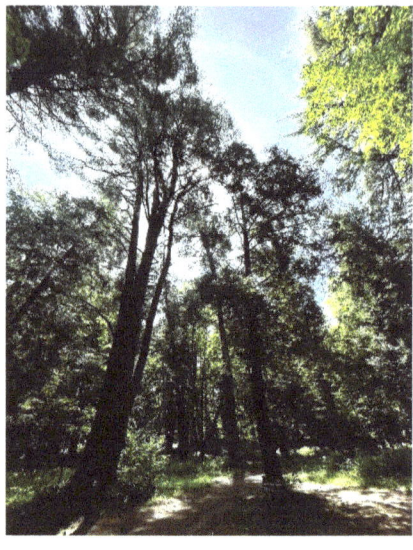
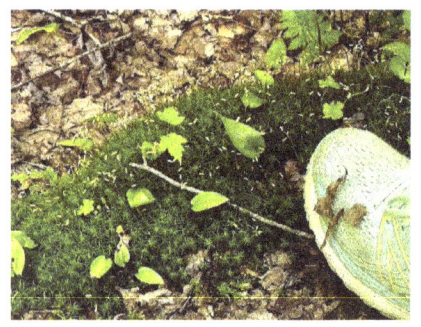
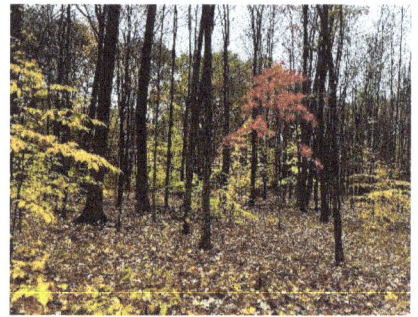
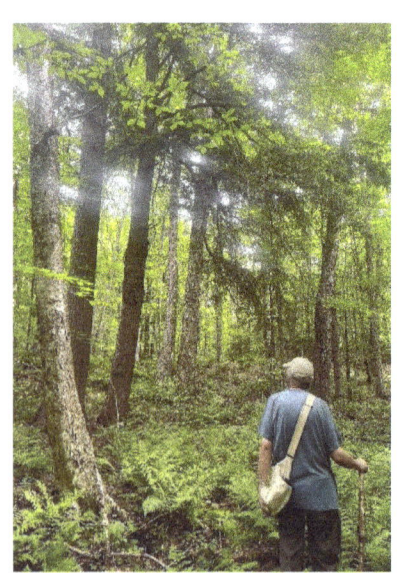
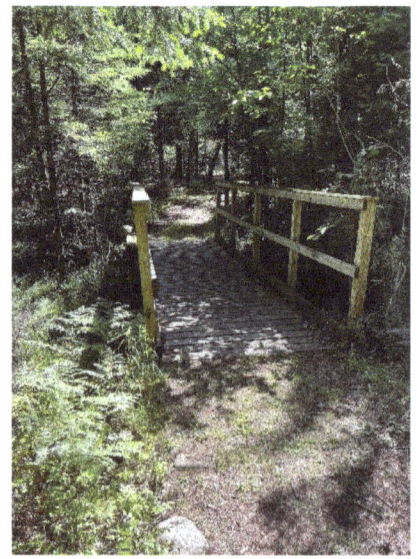

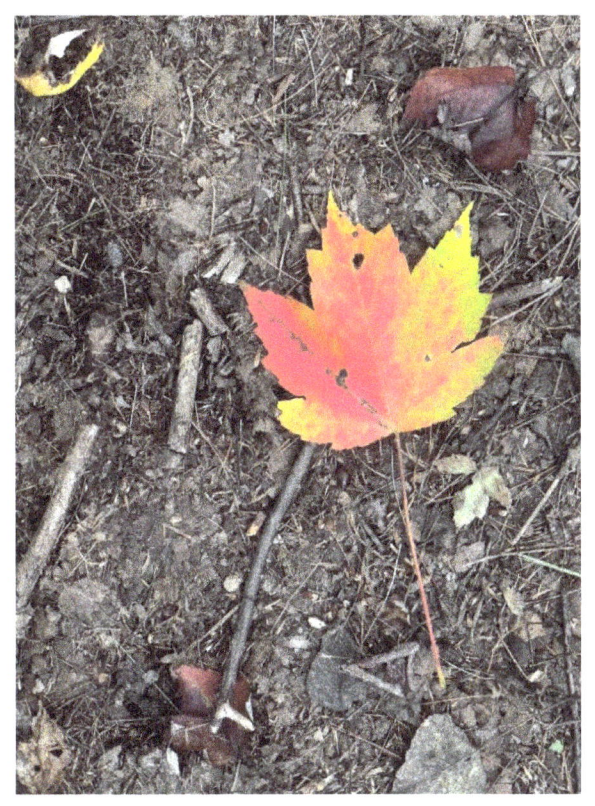

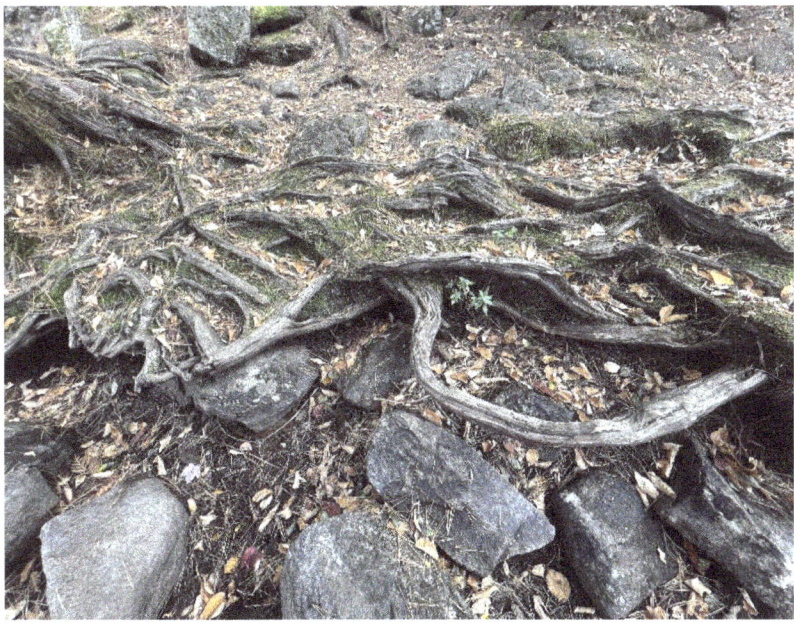

Notice what you are feeling.

Verbalize what you've noticed.

Share what you've noticed with others when you are passed the *speaking piece,* or verbalize it by speaking aloud to yourself or writing in your journal.

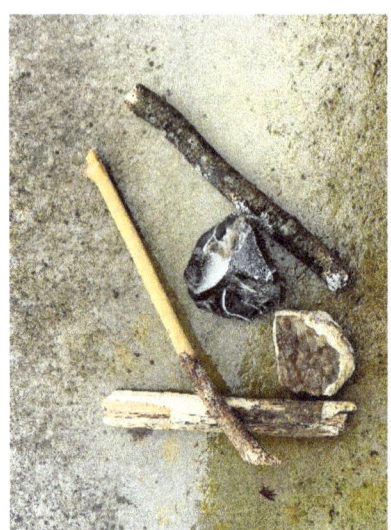
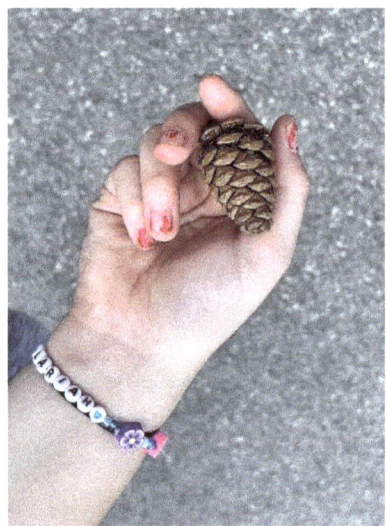
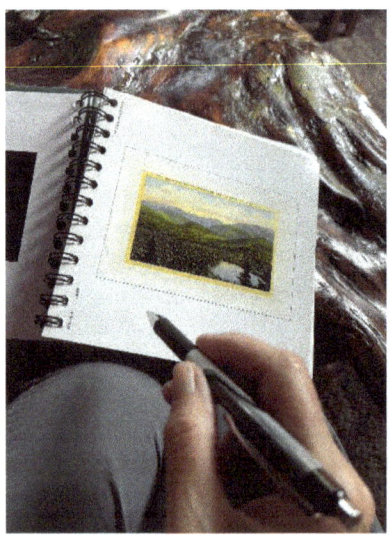

Ceremoniously turn the page or step onto your forest trail across your threshold and be immersed in your natural surroundings. You may add to the sense of ceremonious entry by patting the same tree, (or reading the same favorite bookmark) or touching the same talisman each time you begin a new Forest Bath.

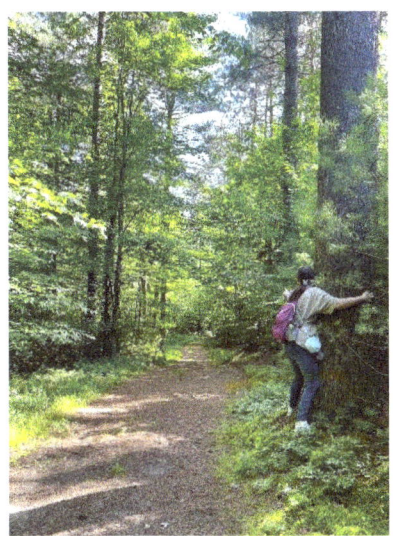
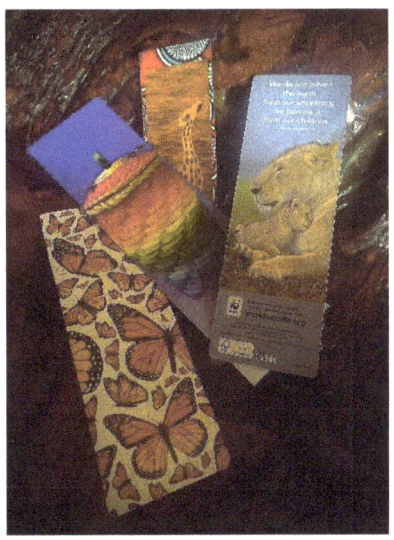
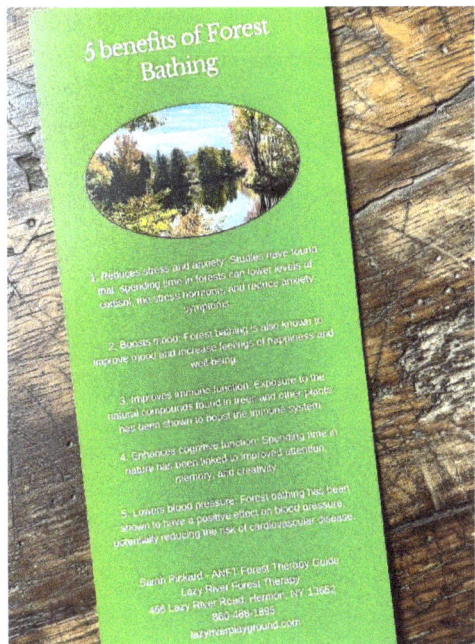

Now turn to these next several photos or walk along your own path for 15 minutes or so as you focus on your sense of sight.

Be especially attuned to movement.

Take your time, walk or turn pages slowly, look up; look down.

Do you see movement more readily than still objects?

Look left and right. What movement do you see of leaves and needles? What of grasses and herbs?

Are the leaves flat green? Glowing? One hue?

Any insects, birds, animals, moving? Water?

Do you see any patterns in the forest?

Notice the change in light patterns…where brilliant, where shaded, where from on high or a low direction.

Is the sky an overcast Adirondack gray? Bright cerulean, pale blue?

Do the patterns wave, flicker, change subtly?

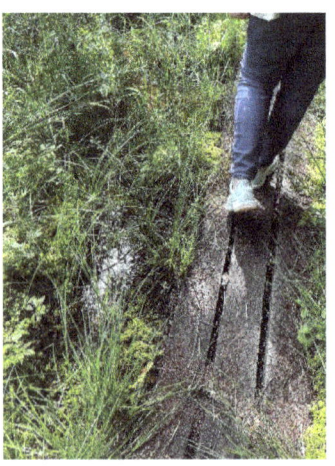 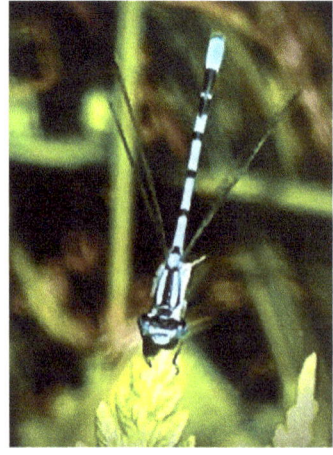

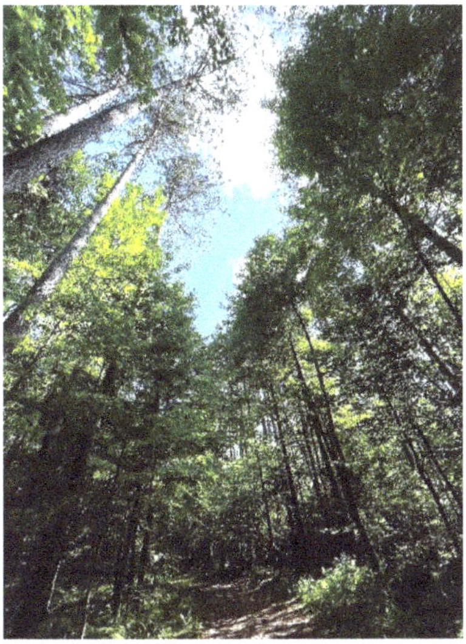

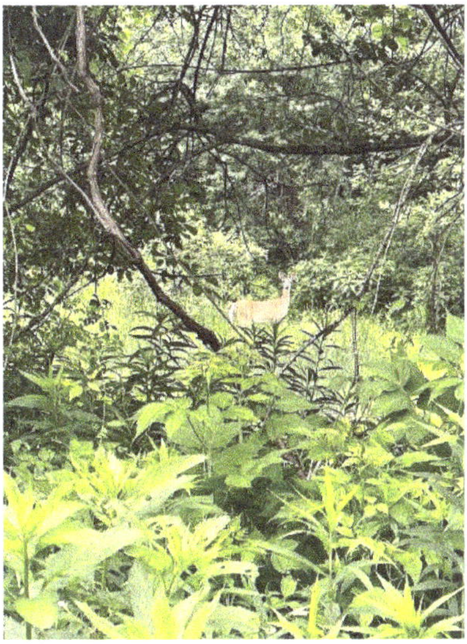

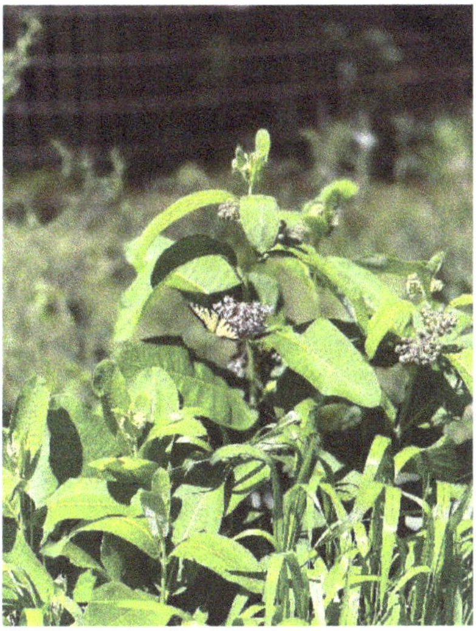

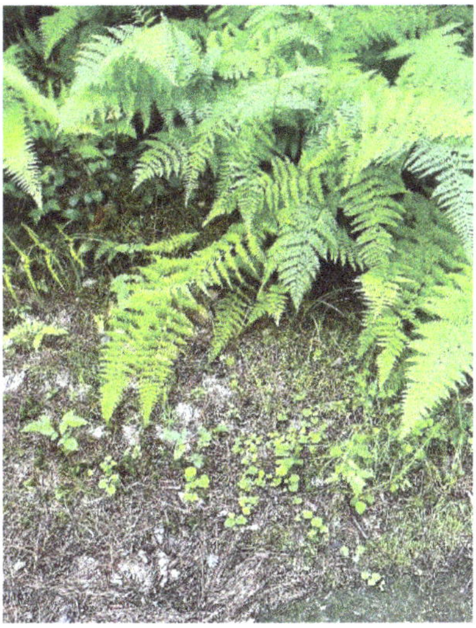

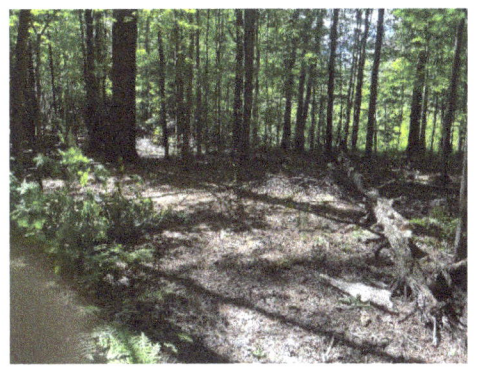

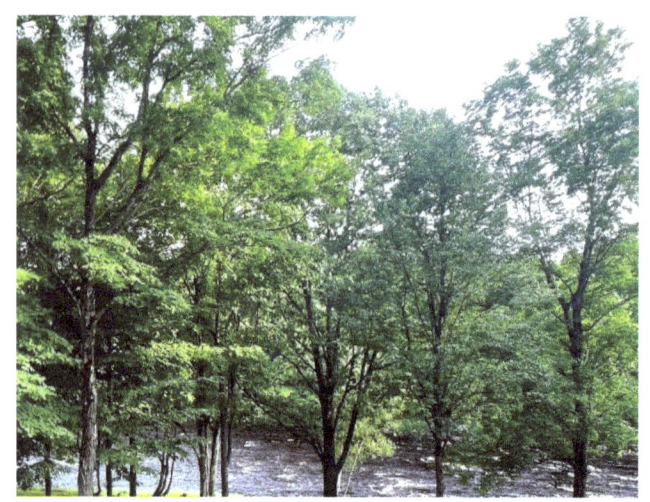

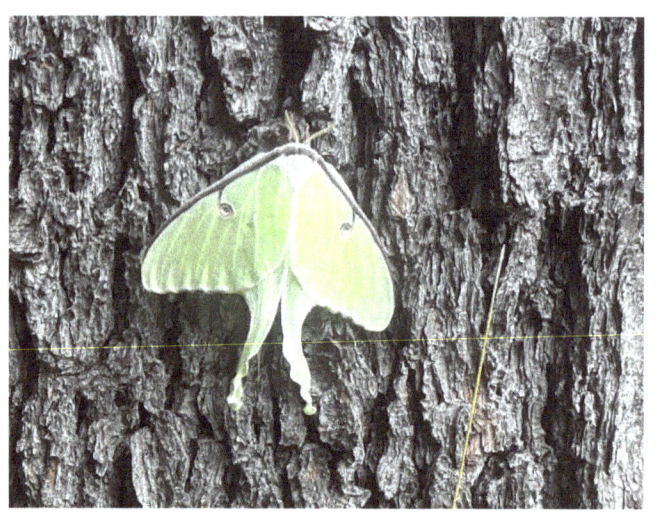

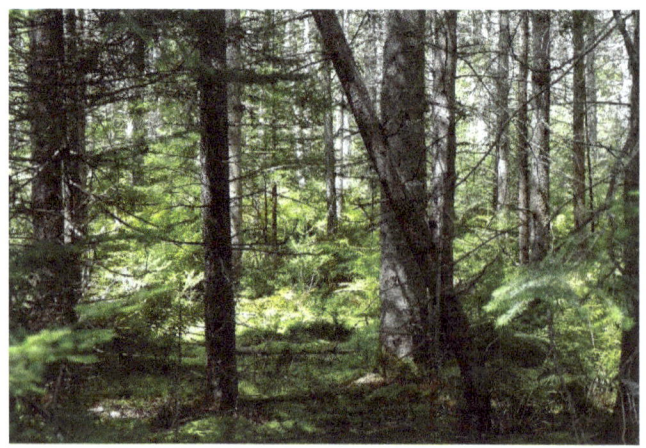

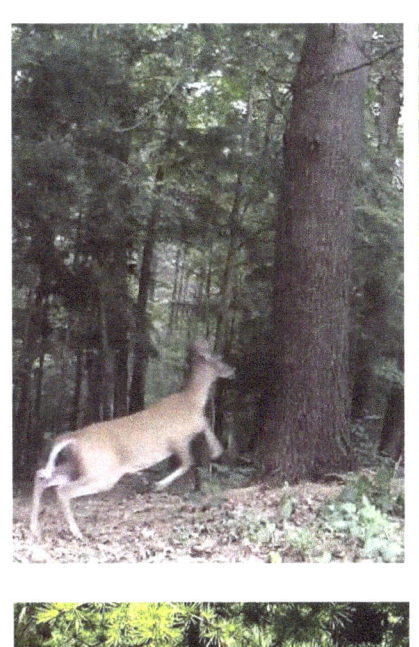
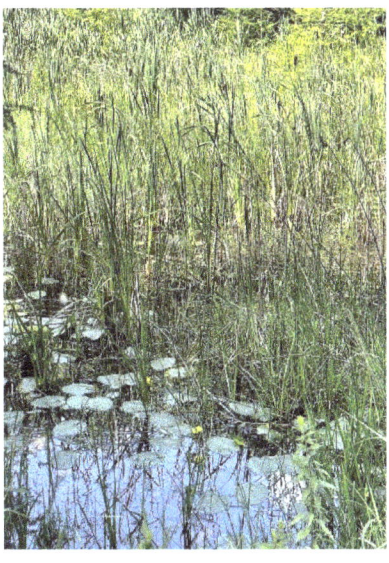
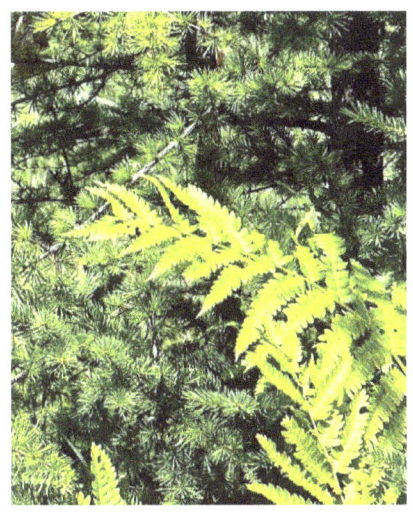
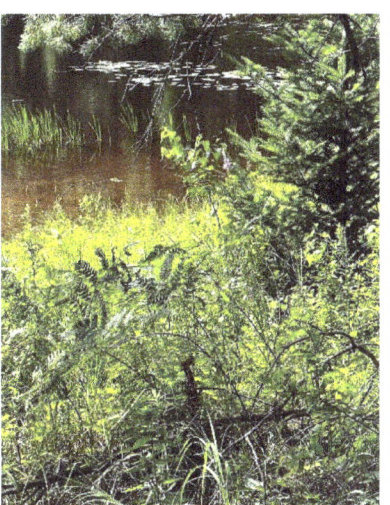
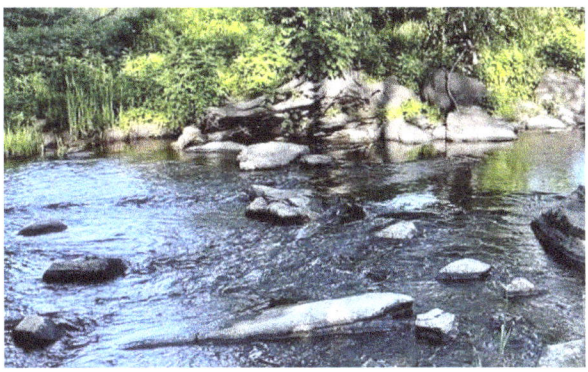

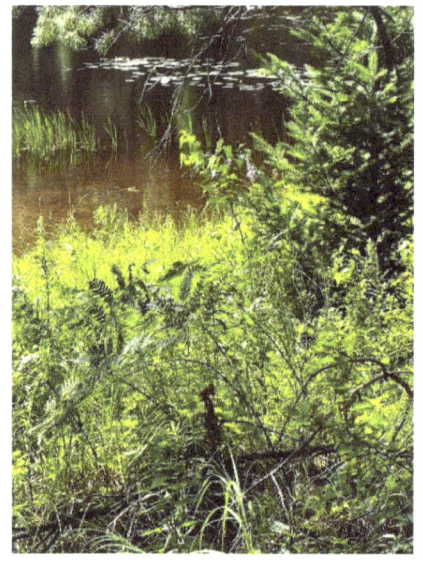
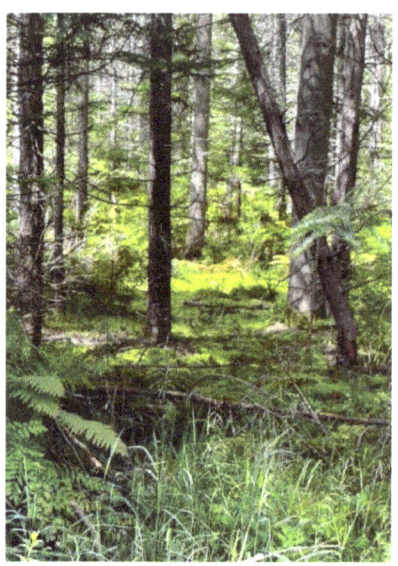
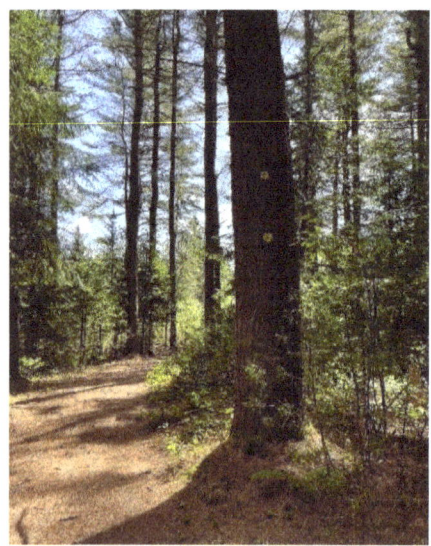
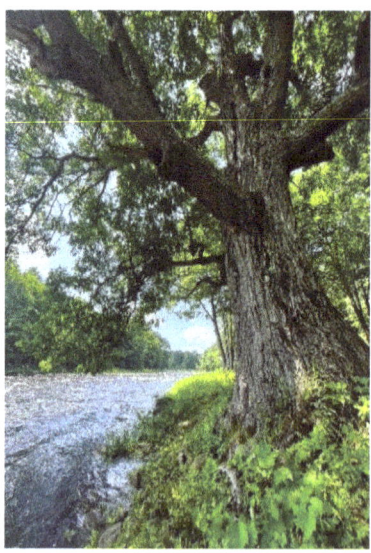

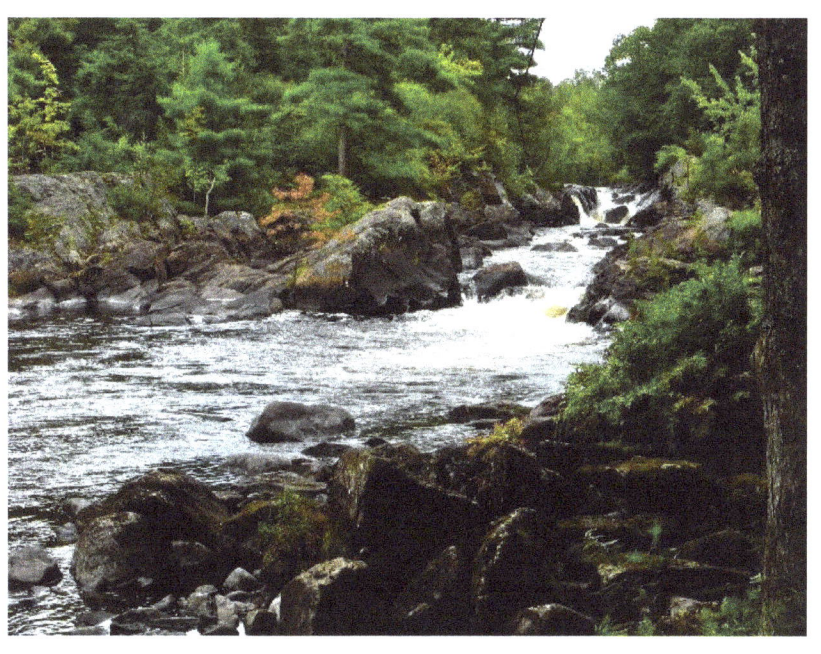

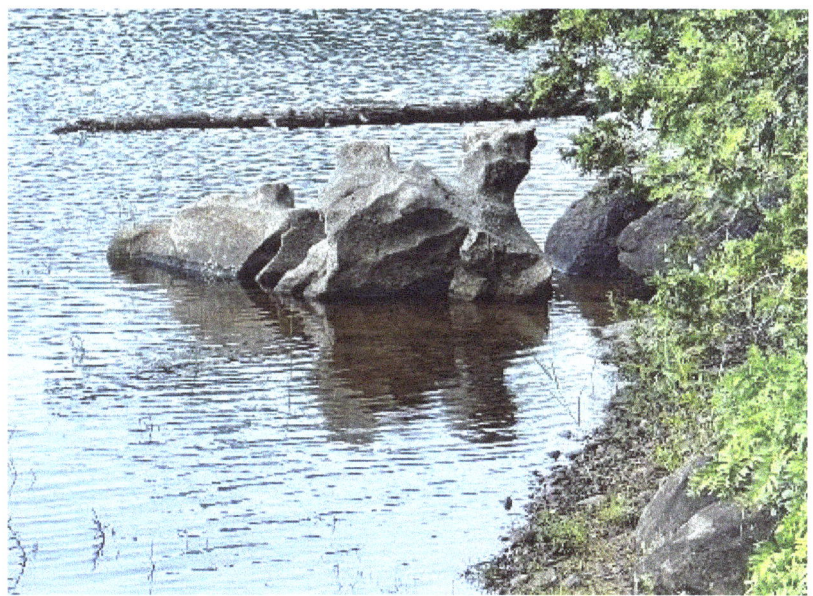

As you notice movement, what of sound?

Do you hear differently with eyes closed?

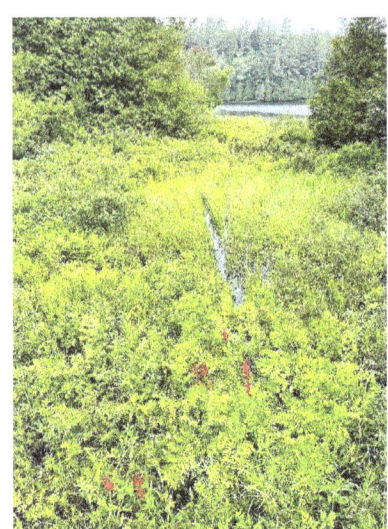
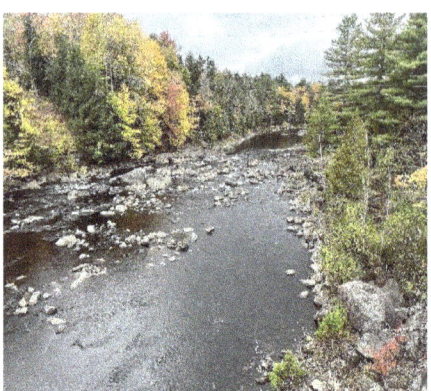
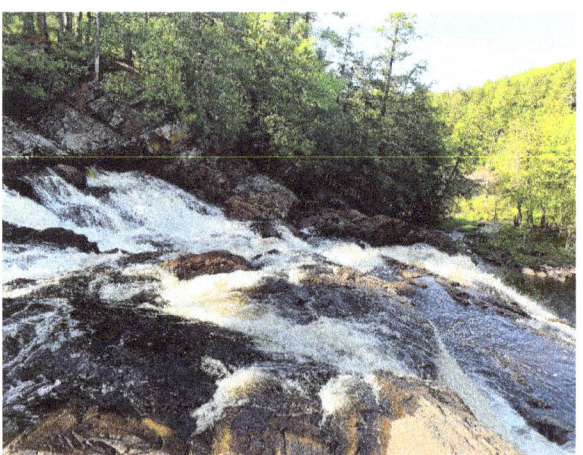
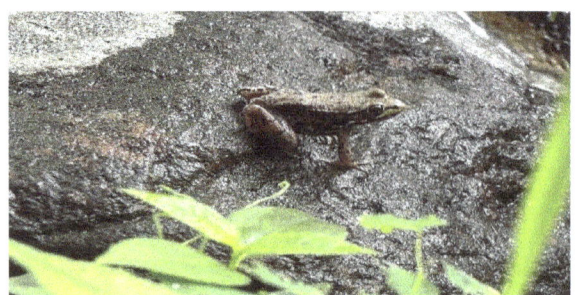

POEM OF THE RIVER BATH

(Holly Chorba)

"Shhh.... QUIET... LISTEN "

shhh…quiet your mind.	Listen to the river,
	rush over shadows,
	rush through passages,
	between rocks and shoreline.
shhh…quiet your mind.	Listen to the river,
	shadow over worries,
	shadow out verbiage,
	between now and never.
shhh…quiet your mind.	Listen to the river,
	push away sadness,
	push out negatives,
	between cries and quiet.
shhh…quiet your mind.	Only the river.
	Sounding in mind's ear.
	Push away, rush, push.
	between shade and sunshine.

SHHH.... QUIET.... LISTEN.

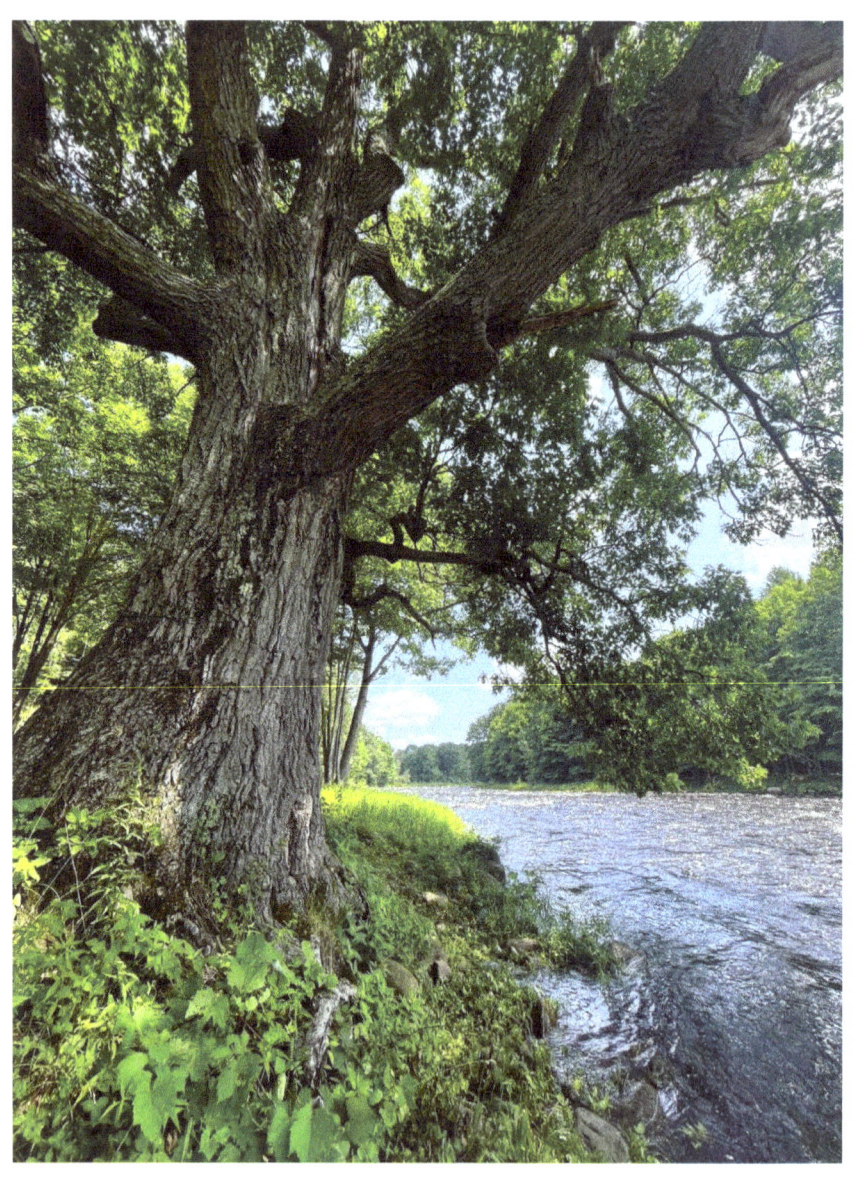

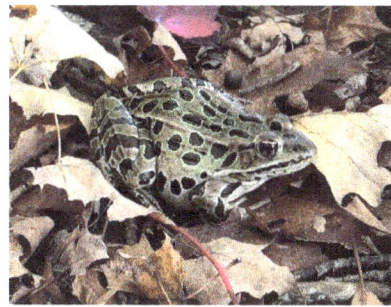
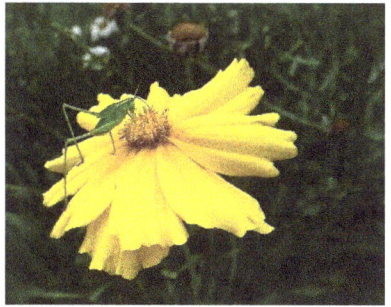
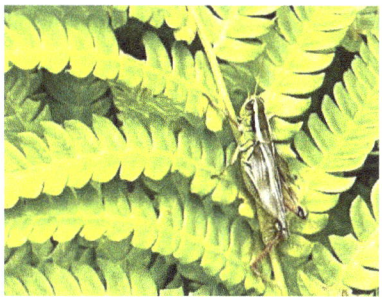

Do you hear vibrations? Your own rustling about or footsteps?

Are the sounds you hear nearby or far?

Are the sounds isolated or in concert?

Be still for 5 minutes or so and listen.

Do you detect differences in pitch? Volume?

Do you hear any rhythms?

Do you hear sounds you know, perhaps the persistent chipping of a chipmunk or bzzz of a cicada?

Listen with eyes open and then gently close your eyelids.

When you are ready, open your eyes and walk on, continue intently listening and looking for motion.

Banish any intruding thoughts of the past or future; bring your attention back to now, here, to the present walk in the forest.

Bring your attention to listening, looking toward what you hear, noticing the sounds and sights of the forest.

When prompted or ready to stop, receive the *Speaking Piece* (or take up your pen!).

Share what you noticed about movement and sound in the forest.

Does listening to others' perceptions encourage you to notice differently or additionally?

Does reading what you have written during other walks broaden what you notice each time?

"VISUAL MOMENTS OF SPRING"

Poem of a Forest Bath, 1996…East Branch, St. Regis River

(Holly Chorba)

Waiting for Spring on river's edge yesterday,
We smiled at a bluebird checking our nest box,
Visiting our bird house. We hoped he'd stay.

We noted a common merganser pair,
Traveling up the river course.
We wondered if hoary ice on the north bank will last till May.

We rake dead leaves from the garden,
Uncovering fat earthworms neath sun-warmed rocks.
The spring sunshine warms us, too. Our work is play.

We count crocuses opening gaily
as sun travels 'cross the sky.
We notice fresh beaver-chews on alder at the south bank near the bay.

We see emerging sprouts; Skunk-cabbage
Greening the river's edge.
Fresh shoots seek spring sunshine, poking through the clay.

Visits by wasps on freshly replaced screens,
and visits near our woods by swallows, robins, turkeys,
even a pair of mourning doves, all seeking a place to stay.

Summer is yet a distant dream,
Winter's chill is still felt in the air.
We walk up river, drinking in sunshine, living the day!

Tomorrow holds what no-one can tell.
Yesterday is gone. Today is all that really is.
Today, on the St. Regis River, we live the moment and love today!

Again walk slowly, deliberately, for 15 minutes or more.

This time, focus on light, color, and form.

Do all the plants have the same color?

How does a plant change from its top to its bottom?

How do the plant forms differ in shaded areas from those in bright areas? Does your skin sense brighter light? Deeper shade?

What plant forms are common?

Do you see only a few forms of leaf?

Is there an interaction of leaf shape and light? Leaf shape and moisture?

Do you see vibrant bright colors, or muted dusk shades of tinted grey?

What colors are like seasoning, sparking up the woodlands?

What color draws your eye?

What objects possess that color?

Are repeating patterns evident, perhaps in water or the sky?

Enjoy the sights of the forest until drawn to stop.

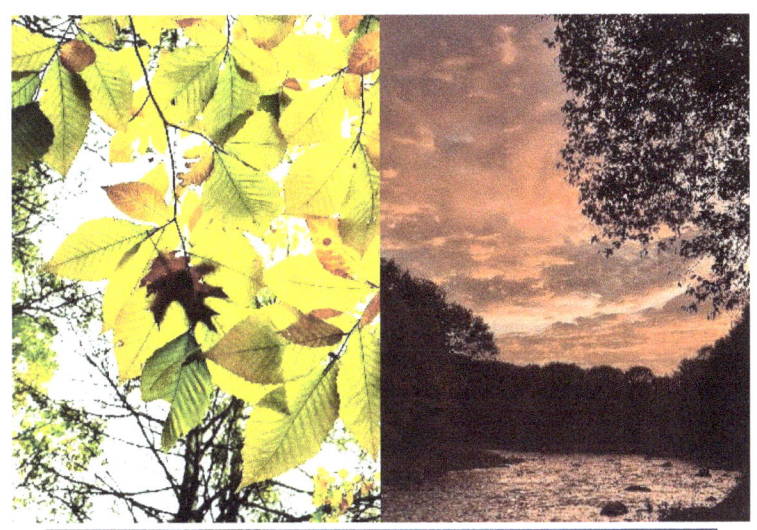

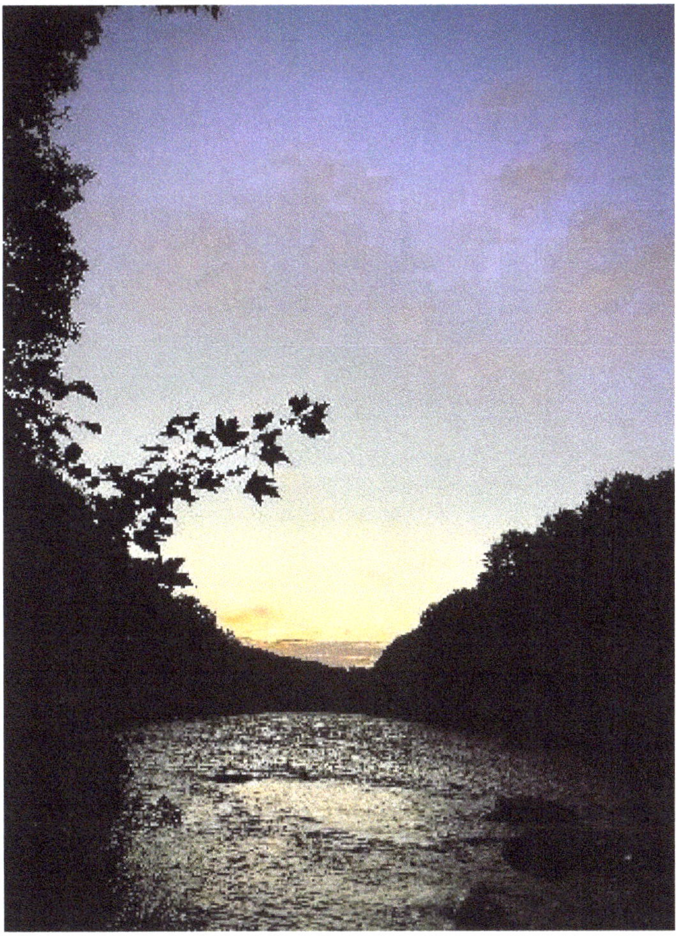

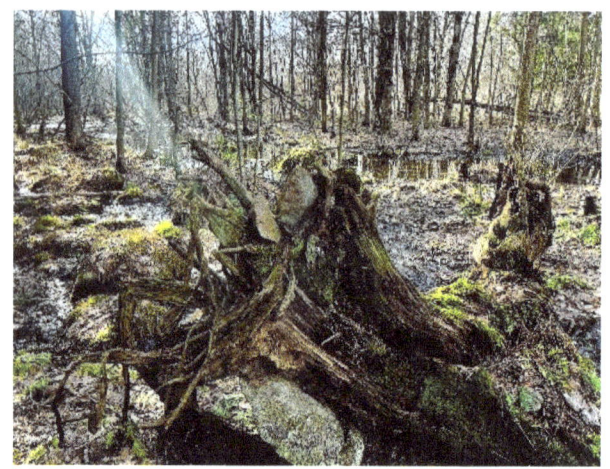

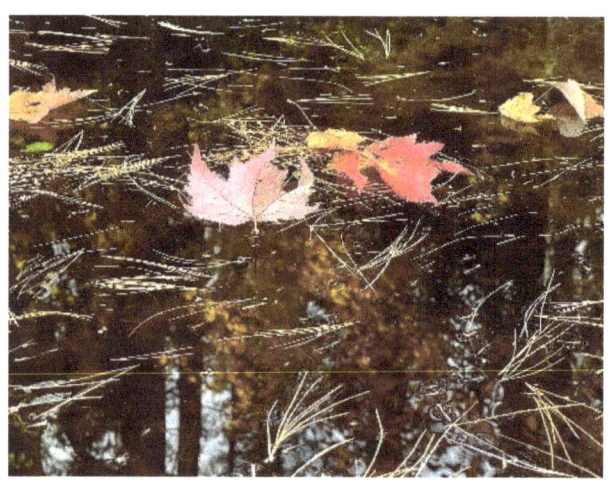

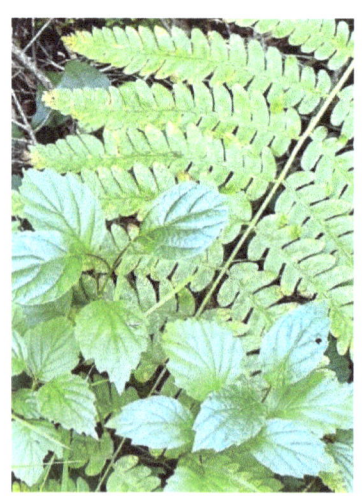
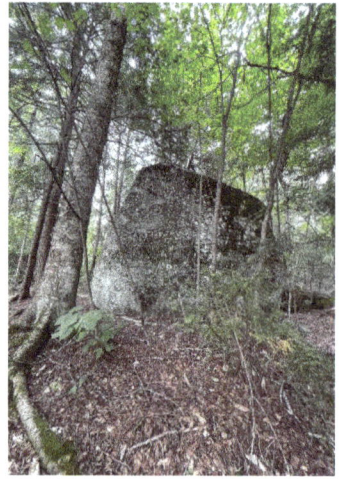

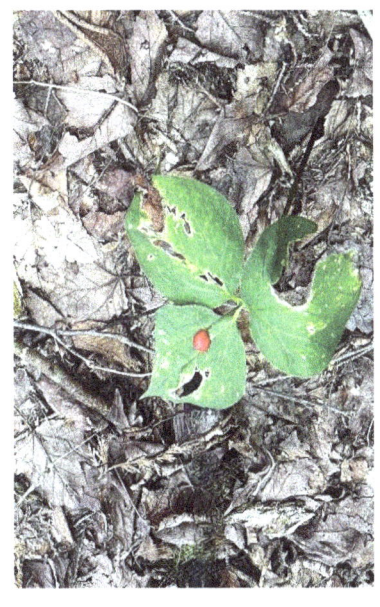
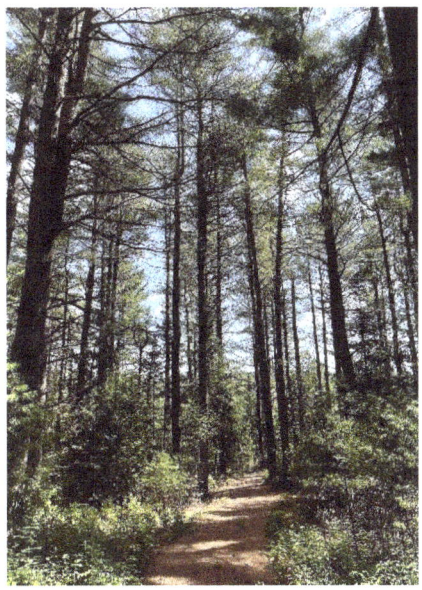
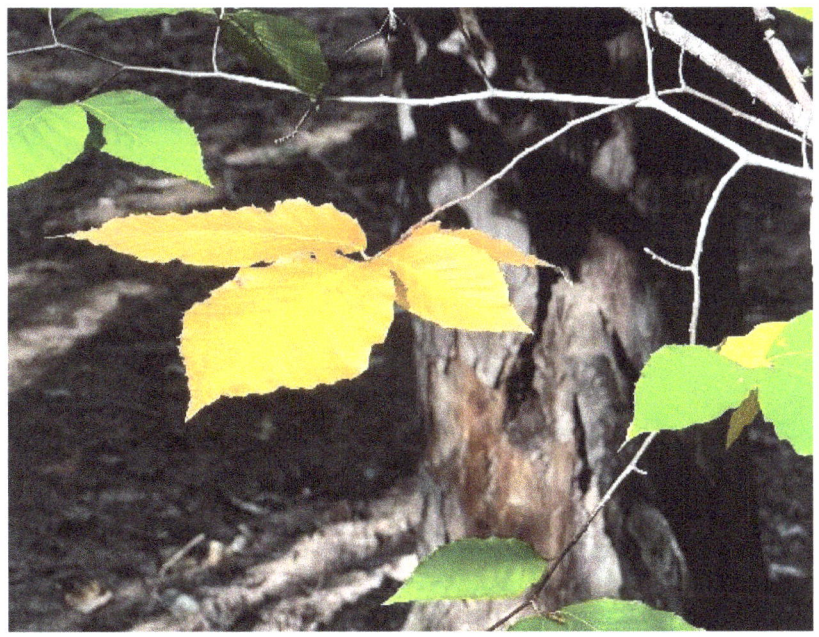

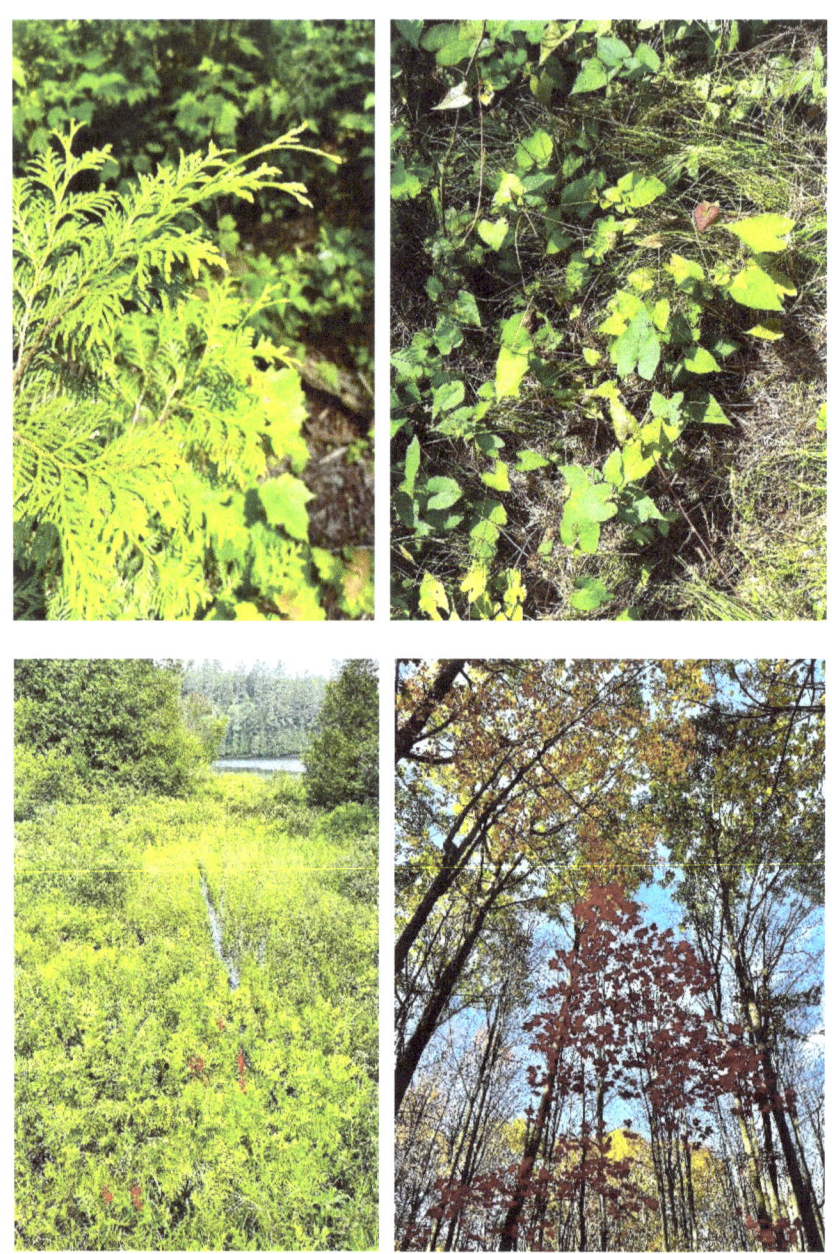

Share what you've noticed in your journal or when you are holding the *Speaking Piece*. You may even choose to speak aloud to yourself. Verbalizing your experience will make it more memorable. Listen to and potentially incorporate the perceptions of others.

Turn further into this book or the woodland. Focus on your sense of touch. Do you sense your weight? Pressure on the ground? Texture under your feet?

Any vibrations?

Do you feel your heartbeat? What temperature do you feel?

Feel the warmth of the sun on your face and the cool of a breeze on your hands?

Is the air dry or moist as you inhale? How does it feel in your mouth? On your skin?

Close your eyes as you touch the leaves of different plants; what do you notice?

Hug one tree, then another. What do you sense?

Feel the various textures around you. What is pleasant, what too rough or grainy?

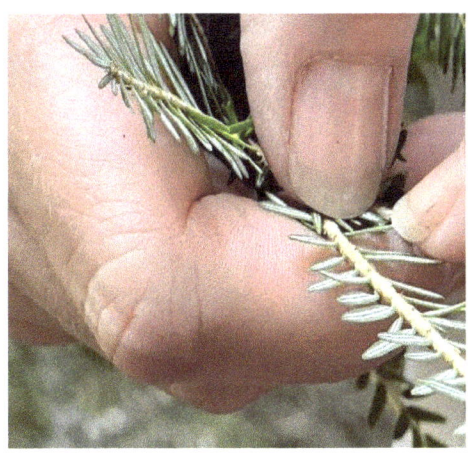 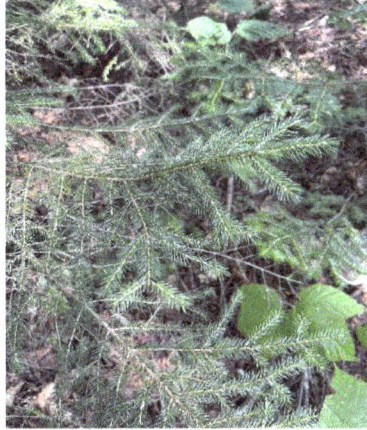

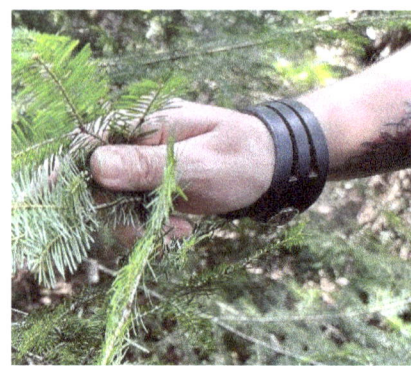
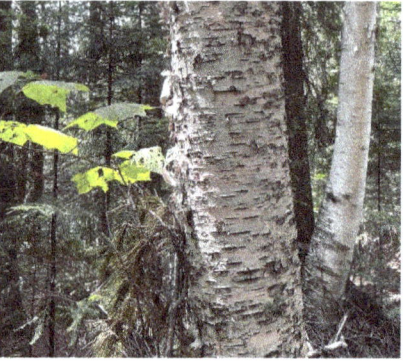

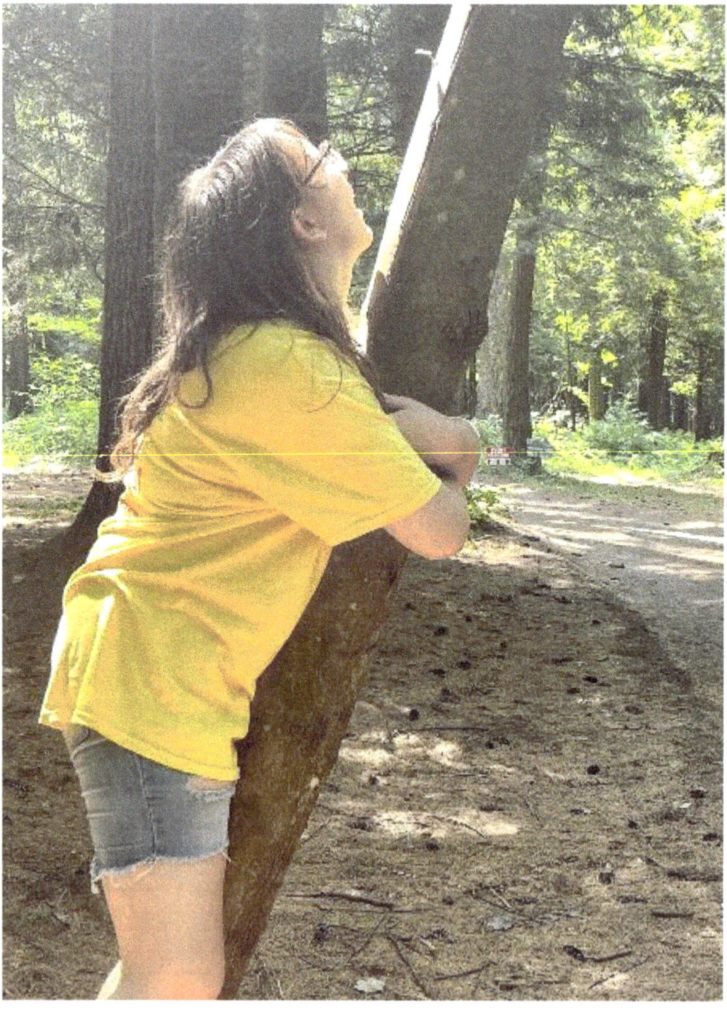

Stand very close to a tree.

Touch its bark. Can you run your fingers down the trunk?

Imagine yourself as a tree.

Can you feel a connection between you and your neighbor?

Can you imagine your roots growing deep into the soil below you?

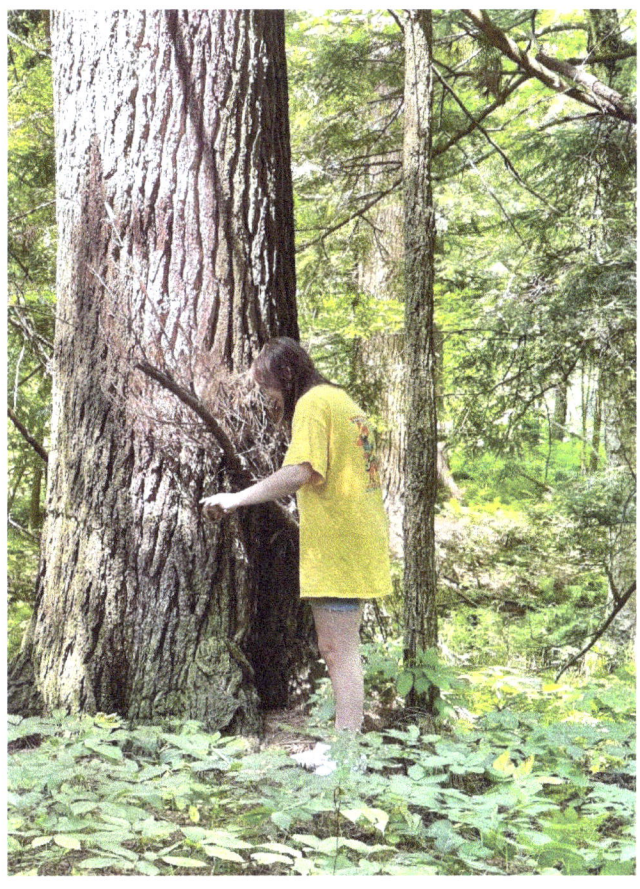

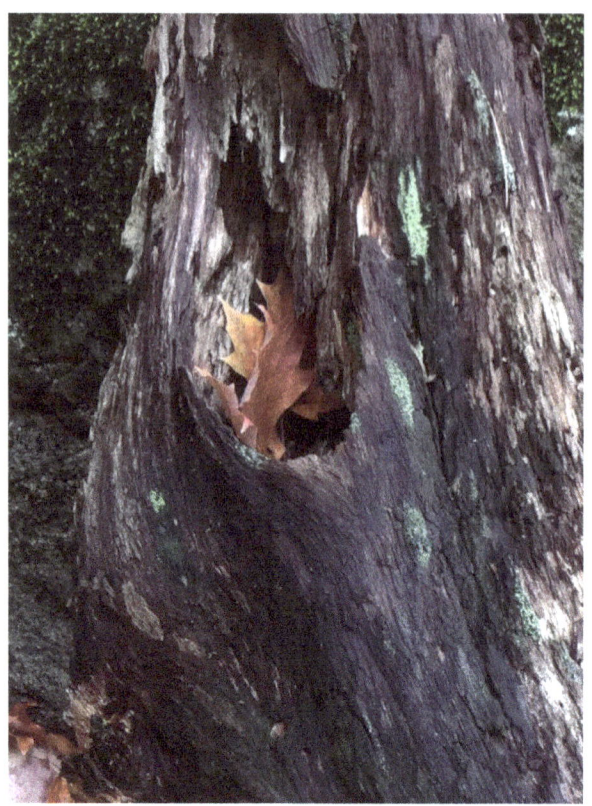

What would it be like to see the subsoil or feel its dryness or moisture?

What roots, worms, or fungi do you see?

What is the texture of the soil?

Reach out and hug that neighboring tree; thank it for giving you oxygen and phytoncides and perhaps nuts, seeds, or edible leaves.

Receive its thanks for tending it, for giving it carbon dioxide for photosynthesis, and for appreciating its beauty.

Can you feel a communion with the forest?

Give thanks to the tree, to the entire forest.

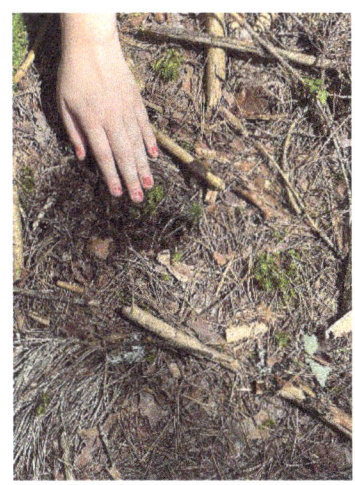
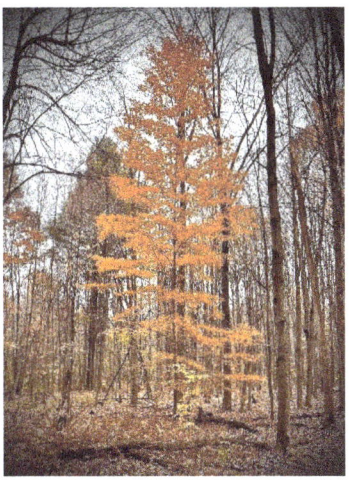
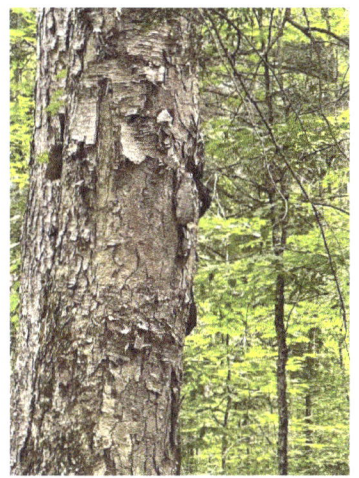
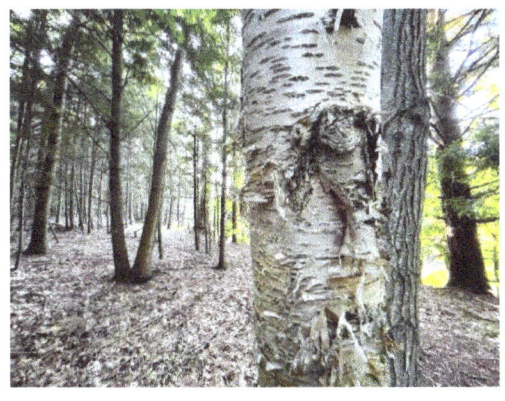

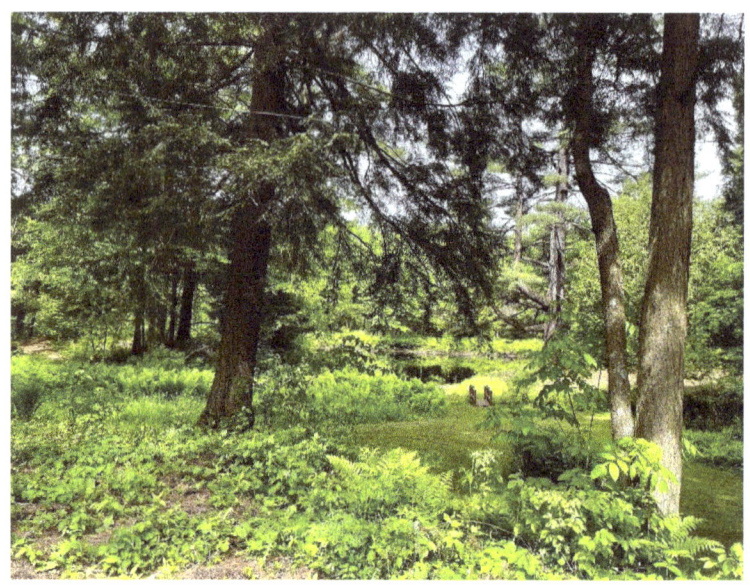

Share what you feel about being immersed with the forest.

As you walk on, notice the fragrances of the forest.

Breathe deeply.

Do you detect delicate floral scents? Mint? Dampness?

Does the woods, in general, have a fragrance, perhaps a smell of "green," or like decaying leaves or wetness?

Is there a clean or sharp smell?

Do you detect the smell of water or the musky or pungent smell of an animal?

Do scents change depending on the level to which you hold your head?

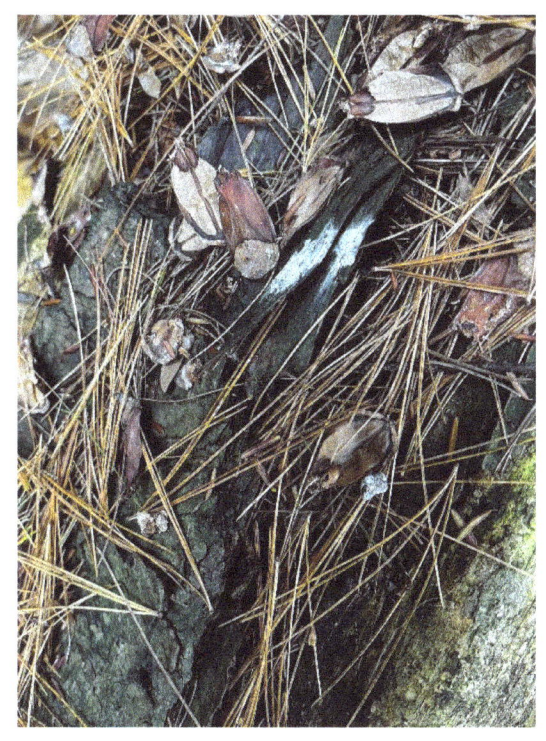

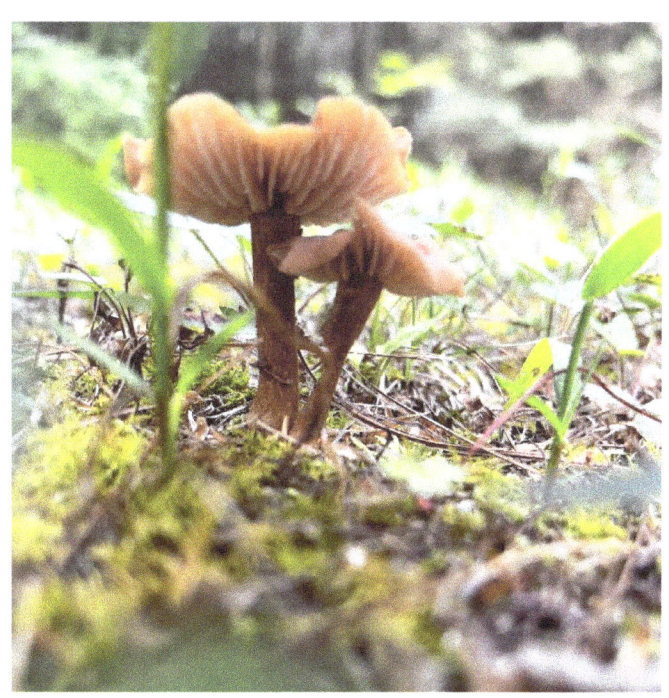

"FOREST BATHING IN THE ADIRONDACK WOODS"

(Holly Chorba)

Walk in the woods with wonder.
Breathe in …hold… breathe out.
Feel the fresh air on your face.
Breathe in …hold …breathe out.
Listen with love to the birds.
Breathe in…hold…breathe out.

Look at the light, playing bright and shade.
Breathe in…hold…breathe out.

Deeply dwell in the fragrance of balsam or pine.
Breathe in…hold…breathe out.
Extend your tongue to taste the pollen.
Breathe in…hold…breathe out.
Sense your position here at the spot.
Breathe in…hold…breathe out.
KNOW, your body here, grounded as a tree.
Breathe in…hold… breathe out.
Relate to this place, to these beings. You are one with them.

Breathe in…hold…breathe out.

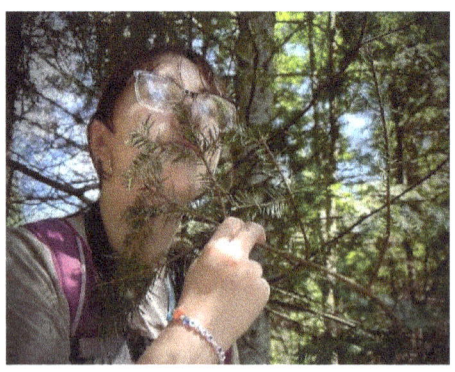

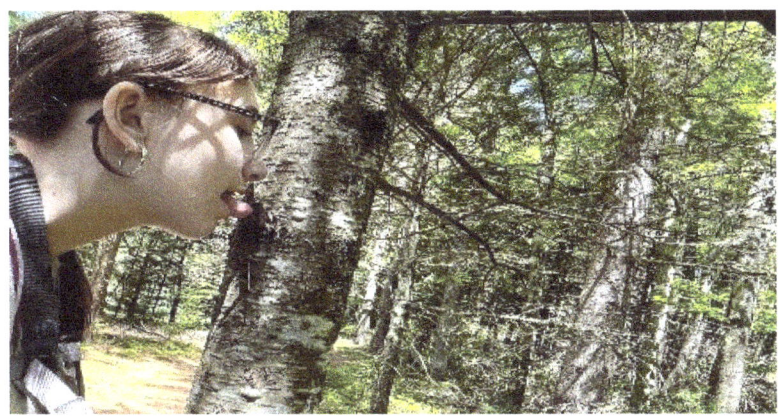

Now, gently open your mouth and breathe deeply through it.

Draw the air over your tongue.

Do you detect any tastes?

Sour, sweet, bitter, salty, savory, metallic?

Hold your mouth near different types of trees as you pass, inhale through your mouth.

Sense any differences.

Ensure safe, non-toxic plant identification and taste a needle or leaf without swallowing.

Share what you've noticed through the sense of taste.

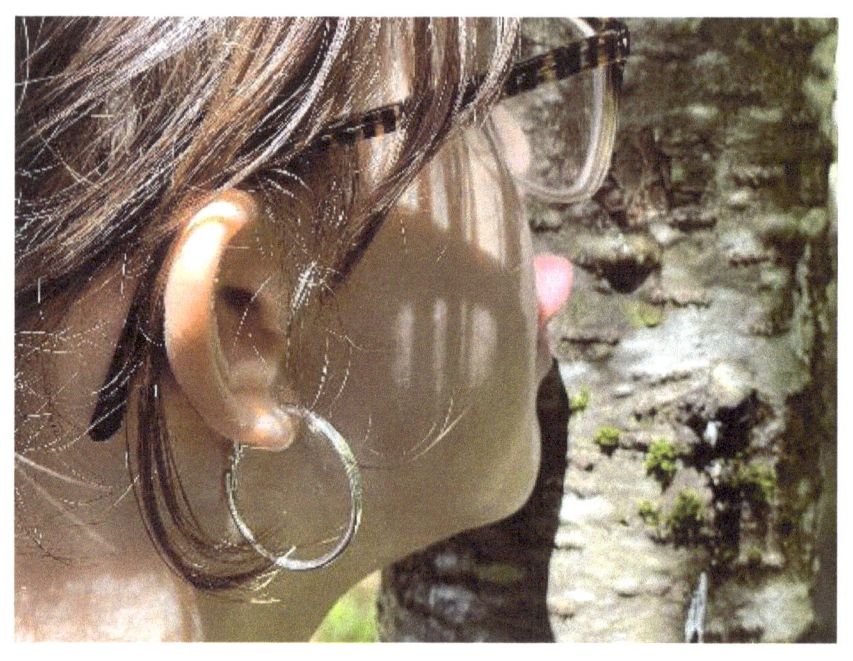

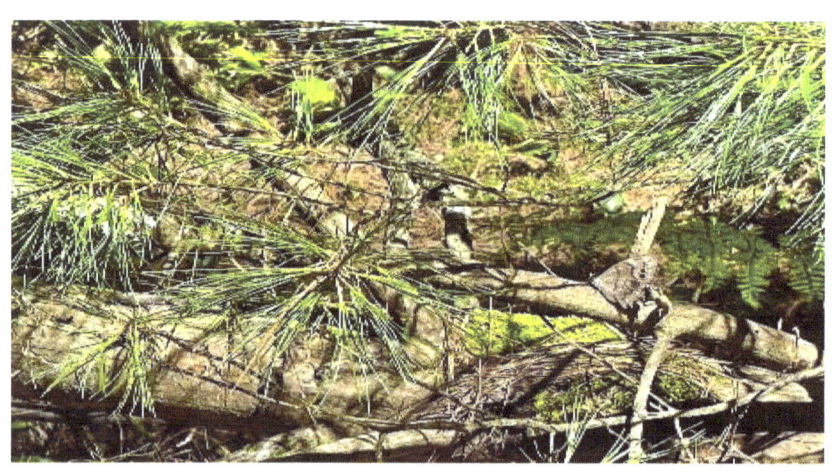

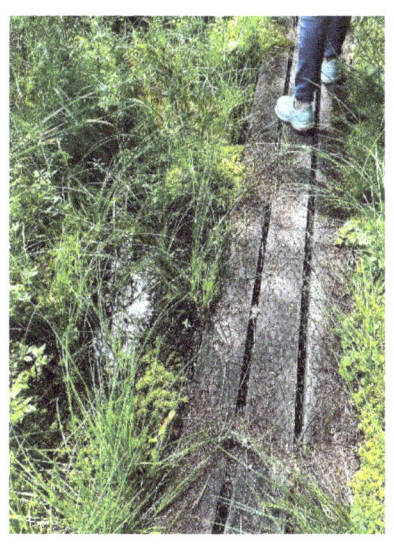

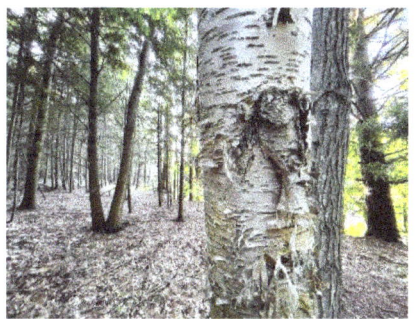

Continue your walk until you come upon a place to be still…a possible "*Sit-Spot*." As you are there for perhaps as long as 20 minutes, you will notice more and more detail.

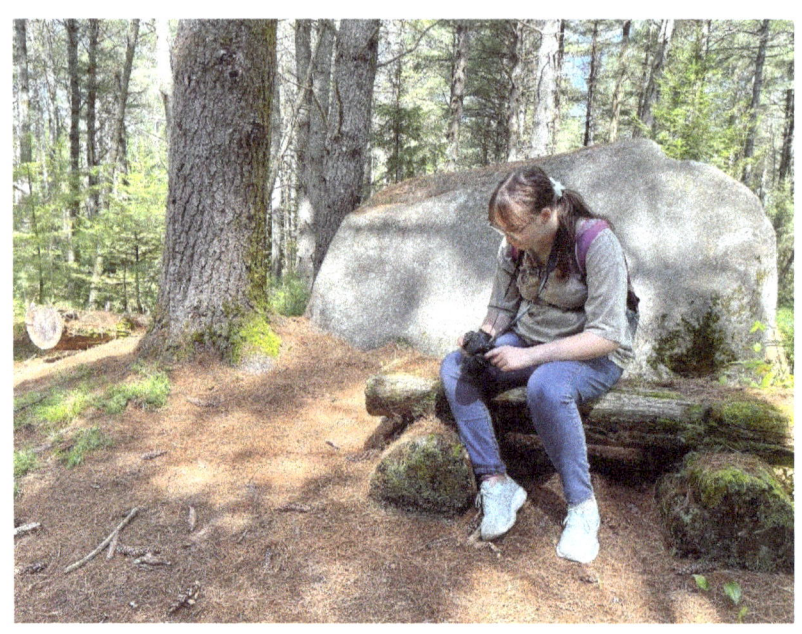

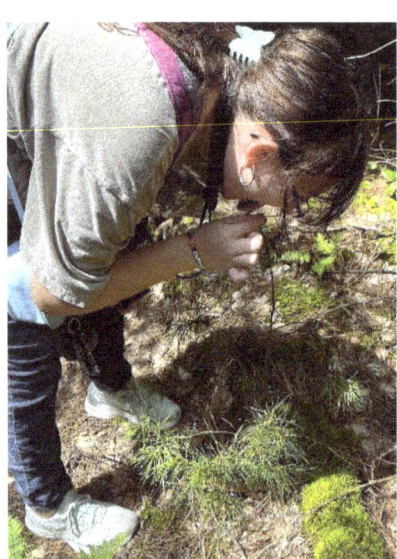
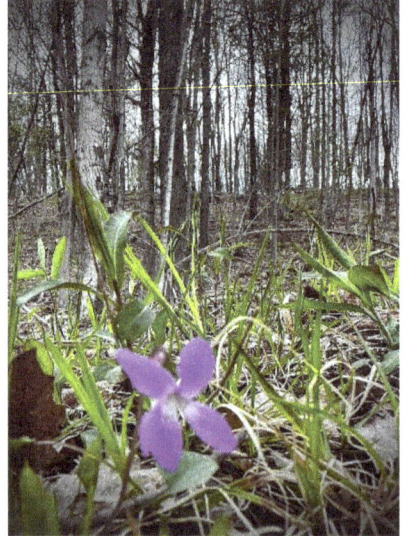

Use your senses: sight, hearing, smell, taste and touch.

Perhaps read the invitations suggested above to guide your perceptions in this spot.

Relax and sense your surroundings. Let the beings of the forest, your garden, or another landscape reveal themselves. Be aware of sounds, motion, fragrances, sights, and feelings.

Hold your perceptions of this spot, breathe deeply, allow yourself to remember it.

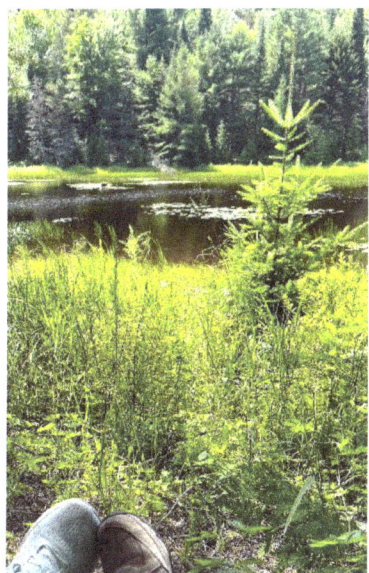 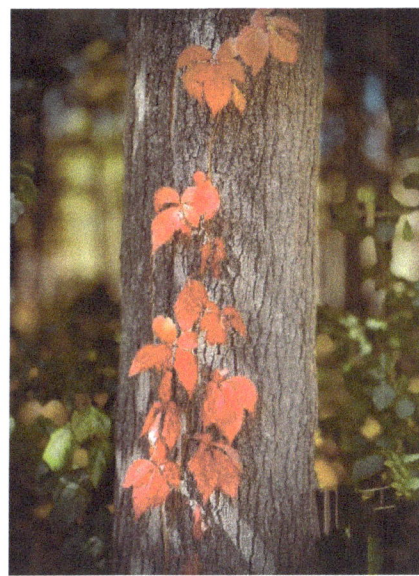

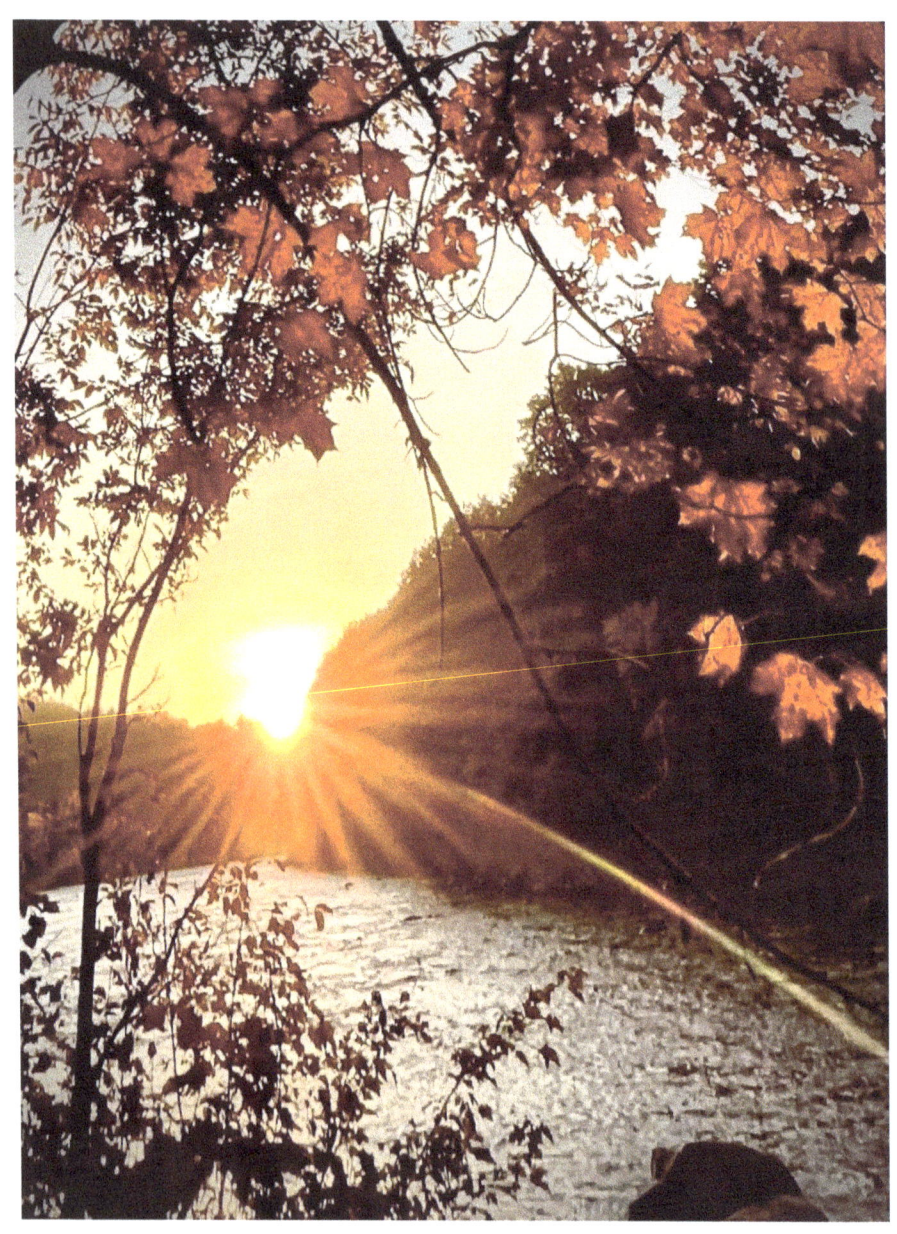

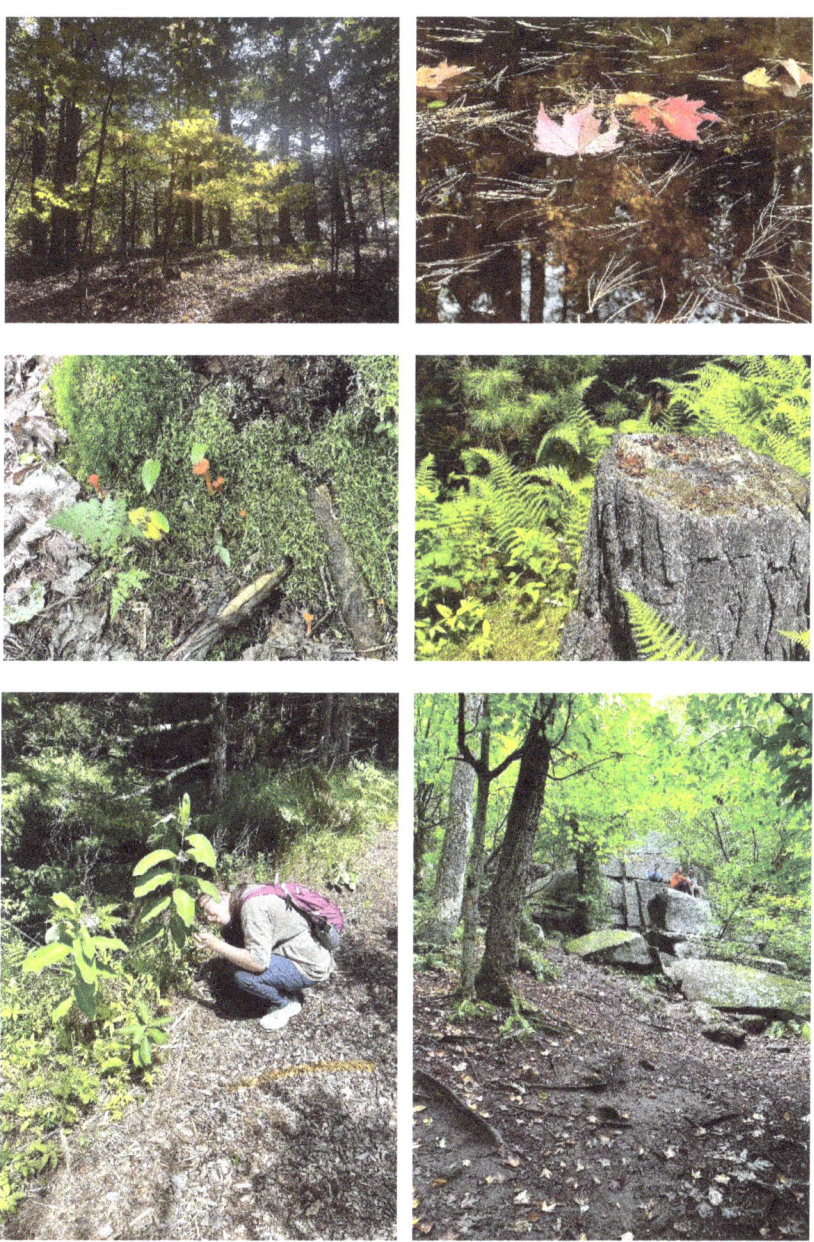

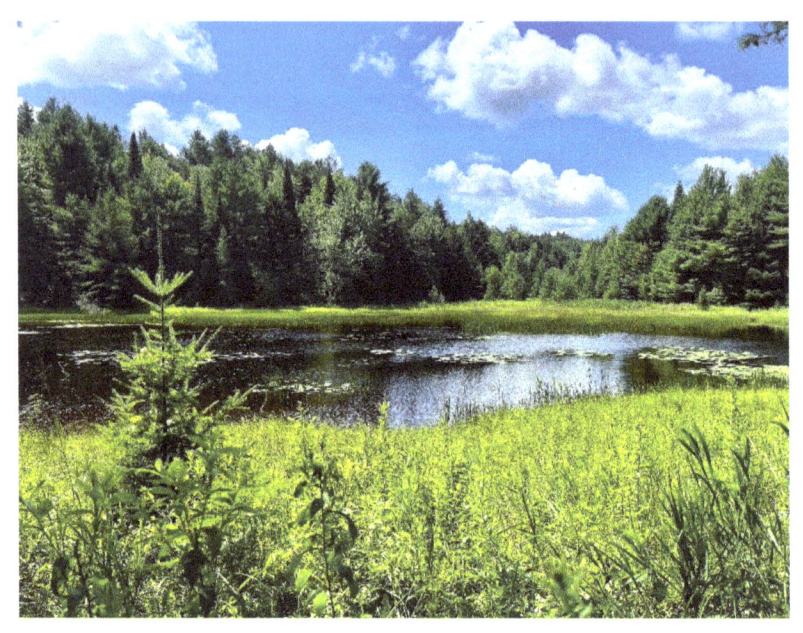

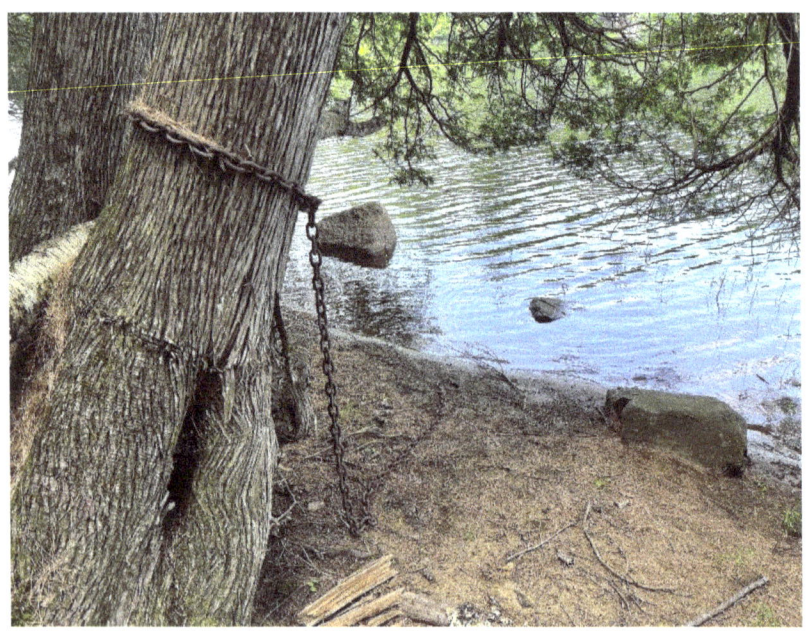

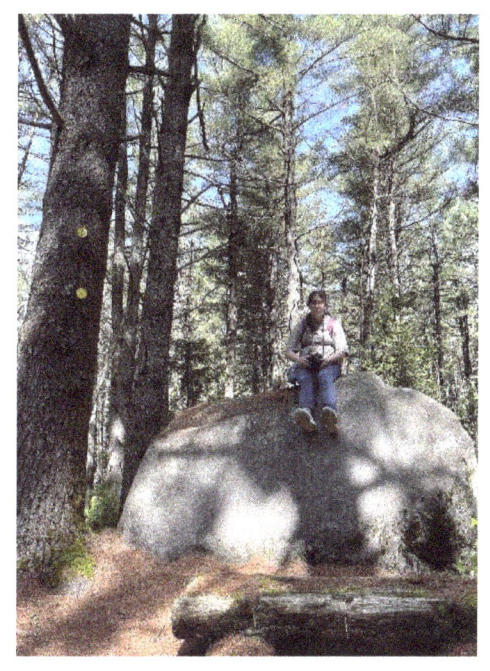

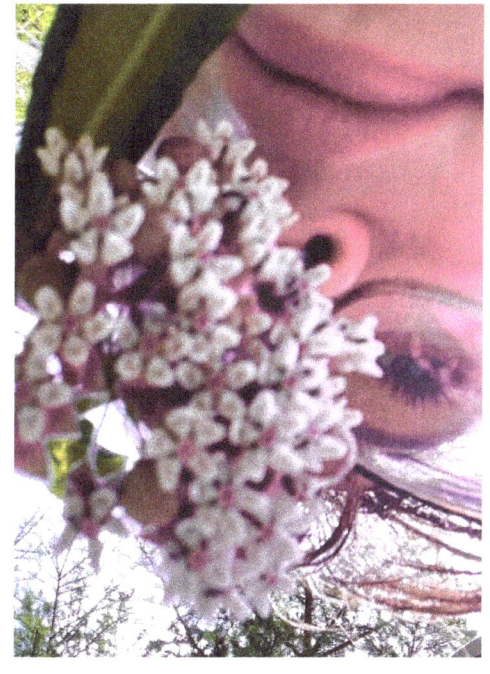

When you are ready, move on to your Tea Ceremony.

The Tea Ceremony is a relaxed sharing of your experience over a cup of tea and a snack. Your tea may be one you brew from herbs that you've collected during your walk if you are well acquainted with what is safe to use. I suggest you bring along a thermos of hot tea (or have it ready at your *Threshold* if you are using the same spot for entry and exit of your Bath). Tea and snacks from a reliably safe source which fit the mood of the forest include commercially available Chaga and Reichi teas, and whole foods such as raw vegetables, fruit, nuts, and berries.

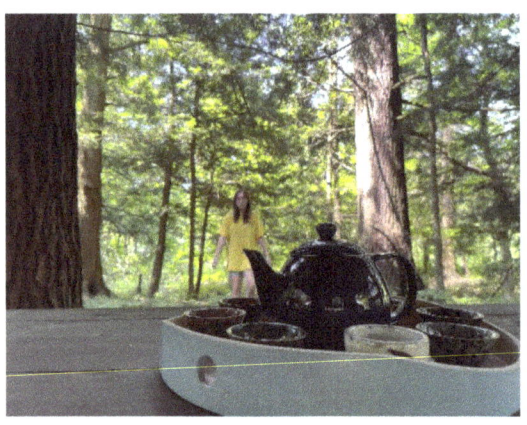

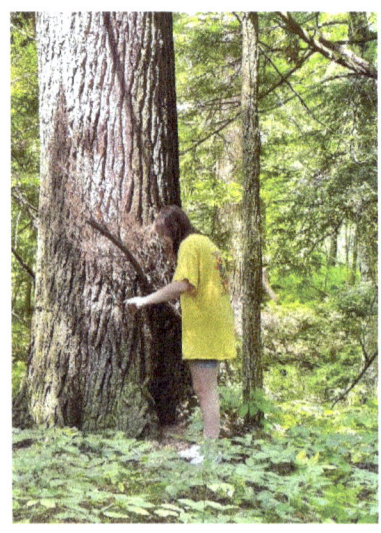

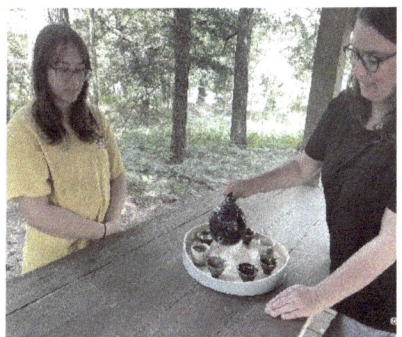 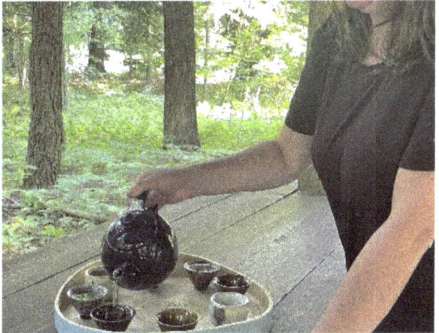

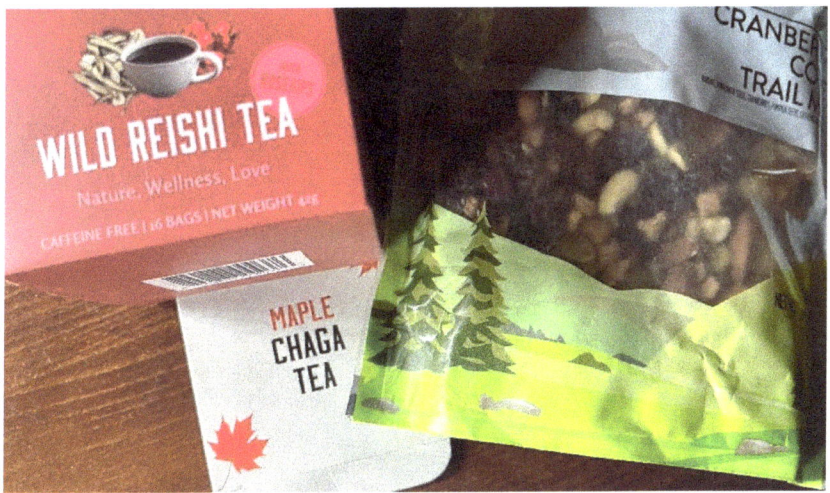

When finished, step over your threshold to resume your busy life. Be sure that you tune into the necessary demands for attention that it holds, such as signing out of trail registries, attending to traffic, medication needs, and attending to those that require your care. Hold the tranquility you've experienced in the forest deep in your consciousness as your secret retreat during quiet moments.

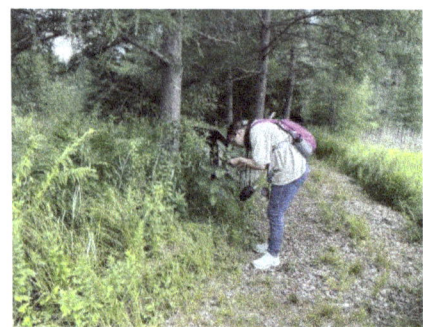
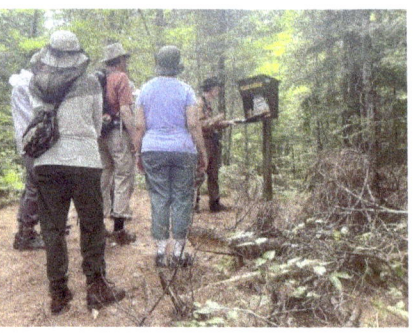
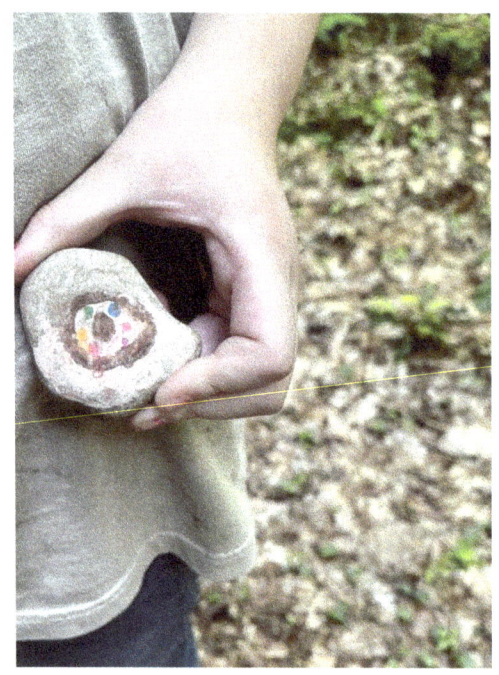
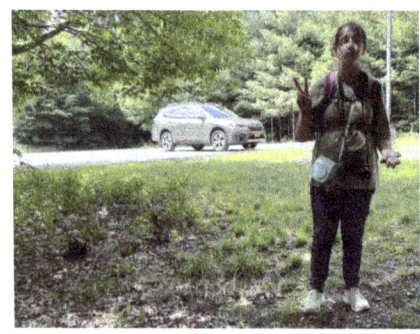
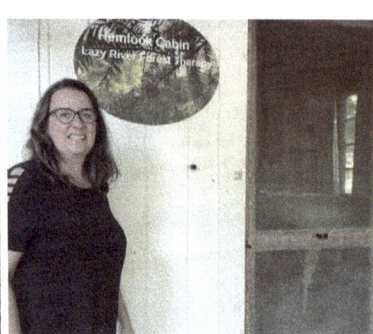

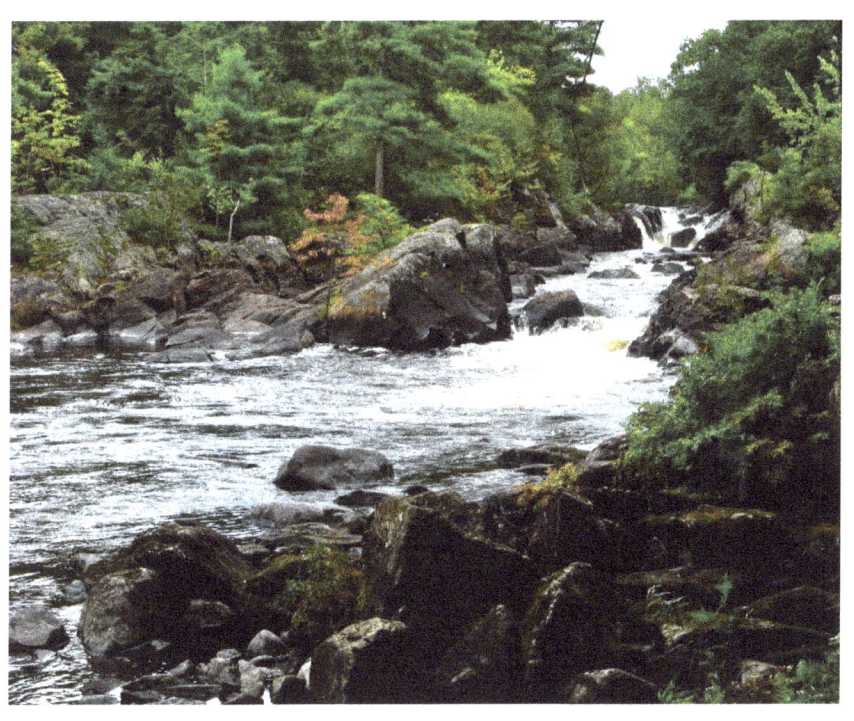

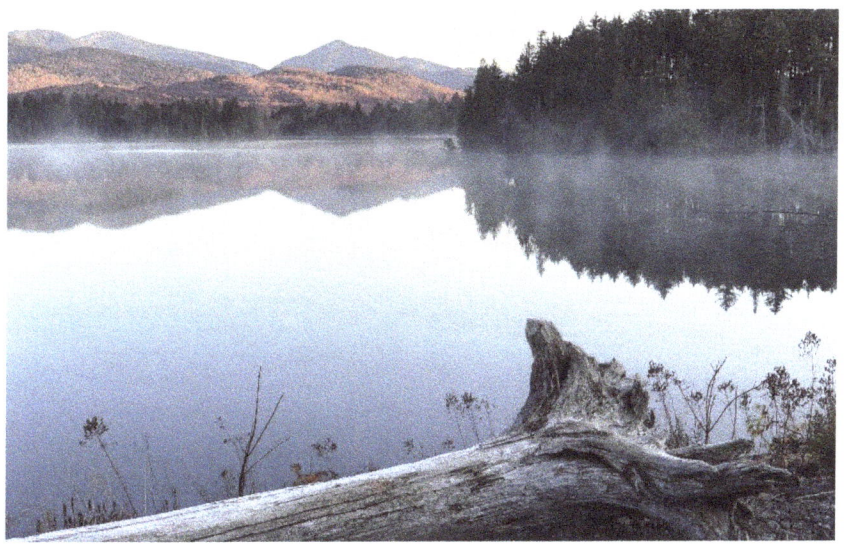

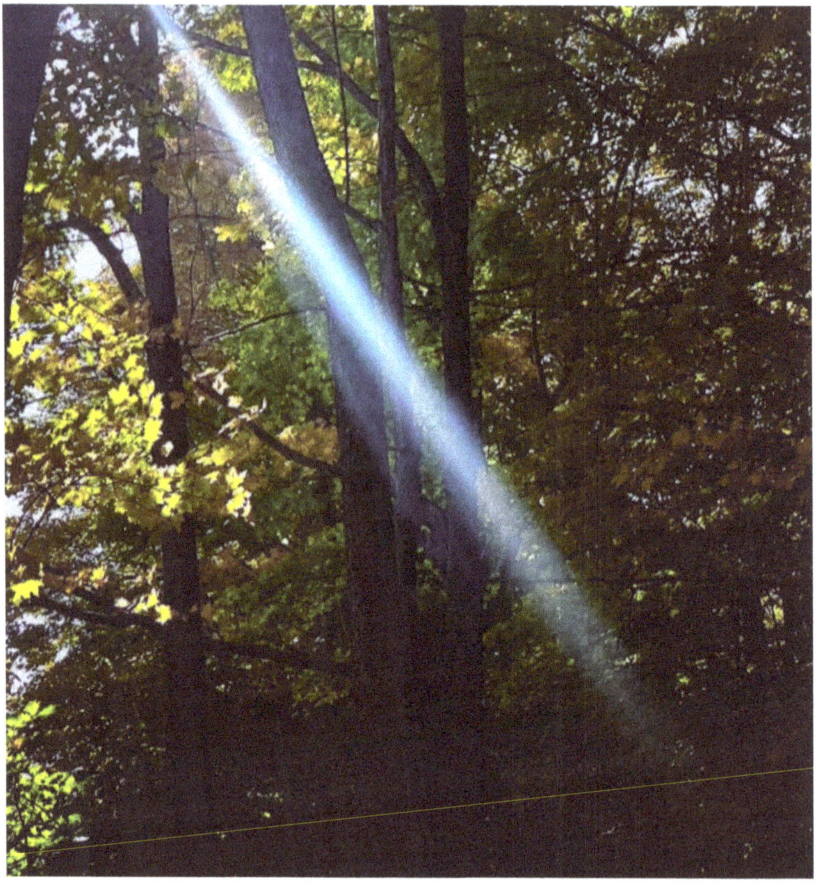

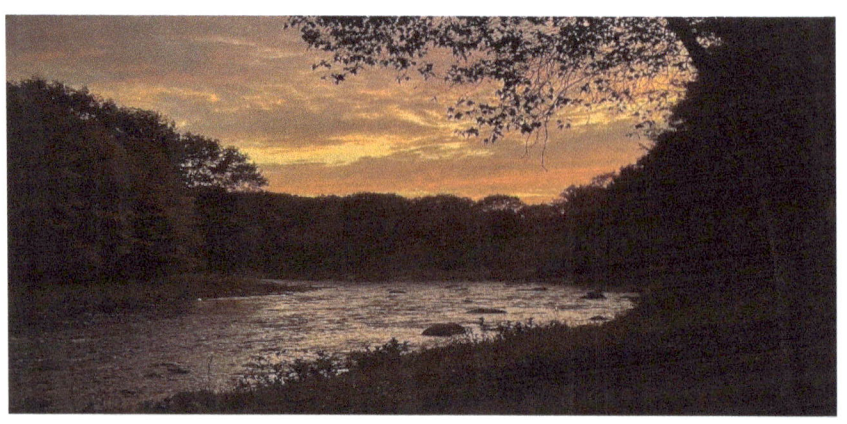

PART III: THE ADIRONDACKS

The Adirondacks (ADKs) have been known as a paradise for hiking, climbing, paddling, and nature viewing for hundreds of years. You sampled that nature viewing vicariously, perusing the photographs of the ADK region in Part II. That sample is only a meager introduction to the over 9,300 square miles of the Adirondacks.

The Adirondack Forest was once known as "The Great South Woods." It covered the present day Adirondack Park and beyond to include all of New York State south of the Saint Lawrence River Valley and much more of the northeastern United States (O'Shea Jr. 2000). What remains now is known as the Adirondack Region of NYS. It is bordered on the north by the Saint Lawrence River Valley, on the east by Lake Champlain and Vermont, on the south by Albany and its Capital Region, and on the west by Lake Ontario, the Finger Lakes, Central and Western New York. Will the area that is actually forested continue to shrink as time marches on?

Since the 1800s until the present day, people have come to the Adirondacks to enjoy its fresh, clean air, serene mountain vistas, and outdoor sports, including hiking, backpacking, climbing, paddling, boating, swimming, camping, and touring. Most of the region of northeastern New York State has been designated the Adirondack Park. Included in its over six million acres are the "ADK High Peaks," 46 mountains with elevations above 4,000 feet, all with maintained hiking trails and beautiful views at the summit, plus thousands of lakes and ponds, miles of rivers, and over 100 small towns and villages. Perhaps the most famous claim to fame of the ADKs is Whiteface Mountain and the village of Lake Placid, the site of the 1932 and 1980 Olympics Games.

The Adirondack region "is, in short, a natural pageant of unusual richness, a feast for the eye and spirit in a time of unusual need." (Edmondson, 2021, p.3).

Today, the Adirondack Park and its governing Article 14 of the New York State Constitution are prized as a model for balancing wilderness conservation, land stewardship, and economic development. This model is perhaps its most valuable asset nationwide. It serves as a real-time experiment in land-use governance, noise, light, visual, and chemical pollution control, and population density and urbanization regulation.

Visitors and residents enjoy overviews of learning about and experiencing the region at the Adirondack Experience (theADKx.org); The Paul Smith's Visitor Interpretive Center (paulsmithsvic.org): The Wild Center (wildcenter.org); and the six state parks within the ADK Park (www.parks.ny.gov). Those who prefer the printed word will do well reading the non-profit publication "Adirondack Explorer" (adirondackexplorer.org). Its 2024 Outings Guide provides descriptions of several adventurous, great trails on which to hike in the Adirondacks; its 2022 Outings Guide describes some other trails, including a bike trail, paddles in the ADKs, and most notably, the article "A Dose of Nature" by Francesca Krempa (Adirondack Explorer Outing Guide 2022) detailing Forest Bathing. There are hundreds more wonderful places open for visitors in the Park. Check out the guides, maps, and literature widely available! Come visit! You will love the Park for its beauty and sustaining practicality. Help retain the ADK Park Agency (APA) to ensure that the wilderness forest will still be here for your children, grandchildren, and all future generations.

Interested in the history of the entire region? The history of the Adirondacks contains valuable lessons for us, lessons that are not too late to learn from and apply.

The ADK forest ecosystem has supported human life for over 10,000 years. Initially Abenaki and Mohawk indigenous peoples resided primarily in its lower valleys and also hunted, gathered, and trapped throughout its mountains. Early Europeans arrived in the 1700s. They too fished and trapped. White settlements came very slowly to the region; fewer blacks settled in the region beginning only in the mid 1800s, aided by the famous abolitionist John Brown. Europeans and Africans both were deterred by the steep elevations, severe climate, mosquitoes, black flies, and rocky soil.

During the Age of Extraction, the mid 1800s, the Adirondacks were over-used as a source of lumber for construction, hemlock bark for the tanning industry, furs (especially beaver fur for the then fashionable top hats in Europe), and minerals such as iron. All these are extractive, non-sustainable purposes and not highly managed. Settlements of lumber camps and mining camps grew. Most of the forest itself was clear cut, and much of it burned. Beaver, elk, moose, mountain lions, fisher, wolverines, and wolves all disappeared from the remaining forest.

The 1800s also saw the more accessible valley areas of the region become sparsely settled. Small hamlets were formed to support lumber and mining camps. Railroads, stagecoaches, and steamships brought those seeking to escape the heat, pollution, and bustle of the city to the Adirondack's great rustic hotels. Lumbermen and trappers, active all winter, became guides in the summer to bring the city "Sports" into the wilderness to hunt and fish. (Kaiser, 2020.)

The human population in the northeast continued to grow. The woods became known as the "Great NORTH Woods," with an increasing number of visitors from southern New York State and the mid-Atlantic region, including our nation's capital. Guides accompanied Sports to the woods to ensure their safety and proper provisioning; the ADK Guide Boat was developed to transport them; small remote camps with primitive lean-tos were built to shelter them.

An increasing number of people began to seek out the nature and wilderness of the Adirondacks just to refresh their spirits. Most such camps have gotten lost in history, but the "Philosophers' Camp" was "preserved" in the famous painting by William James Stillman. It was the primitive escape for Ralph Waldo Emerson, James Russell Lowell, and several other well known doctors, scientists, and lawyers in the 1850's. There, "Emerson is moved by his immersion in the virgin forest and responds to it in a deeper, more spiritual way."

(https://concordlibrary.org/special-collections/emerson-celebration/Em_Con_80).

This attitude grew as evidenced by the Naturalist Movement, concurrent with and balancing the Gilded Age of the late 1800's.

The rich and famous families, including the Durants, Morgans, Vanderbilts, Carnegies, Webbs, Whitneys, Rockefellers, and Posts, financed "Great Camps" to serve as summer retreats for their guests, as many as 99 at one time. Architects W.W. Durant, William Coulter, W. Distin, and Robert Robertson designed rustic yet luxurious enclaves. These designs were later modified for lodges across the country, including several lodges at our now designated

National Parks. In the ADKs several such "camps" also served to preserve vast acreages, even entire mountainsides. In doing so, they isolated beautiful tracks of forests, streams, ponds, and lakes. They also attracted many guests and visitors, supplied employment opportunities for hunting and fishing guides and for small communities that supplied other services and goods such as caretaking, cleaning, and provisioning of milk, meat, vegetables, and flour. Several such "Great Camps" are now owned by the State of New York and serve similar functions as an important part of the State's tourist economy.

Also, in the mid-1800s, people began to be concerned with deforestation. Millions of acres had been stripped of trees; game had become rare; fires on areas covered with dead branches from removed logs were common; several rivers were clogged with logs and silt. People recognized that the watershed of New York City was in danger. The Adirondack Forest Preserve was established in 1885 as a response to those concerns, as well as to the concern that the natural beauty of the area was in danger. (Flynn, 2013, p.8)

The Adirondack Park itself was established in 1892 to protect its 6 million acres as "forever wild." The area is bigger than the parks of Yellowstone, Yosemite, Grand Canyon, Glacier, and the Great Smokey Mountains National Parks combined. It encompasses more than 3,000 lakes, 30,000 miles of rivers and streams, patches of old growth forest, and some globally unique wetlands (a2acollaborative.org/protected-areas.html). It is a state park with no entry gates or fees, 120 included hamlets and 9 villages, and 1.1 million acres of designated "Wilderness" (State of the Park, Adirondack Council, 2023, p.4).

The early 1900s saw thousands more people flocking to the Adirondacks to restore their physical health in the clean, cold ADK air. Henry L. Trudeau, seeking relief from his own tuberculosis, developed the Trudeau Laboratory in the 1880s. "By the 1890s, Trudeau's Adirondack Cottage Sanitarium at Saranac Lake was the world's foremost center for the study of the disease," and hundreds stayed at the cottages seeking cure. (Schneider, p.168,1998).

Martha Reben was one of those seeking relief from TB. Her health was not recovered by a 3 year, 6 month stay in the village of Saranac Lake, so she answered a wanted advertisement by ADK guide Fred Rice to "go into the woods for the summer." She went, improved, and continued to live at the small summer camp on Weller Pond in the ADK woods for years. After 10 years, her x-rays confirmed she'd been cured. Years after that, she wrote that stays in the forest bestowed upon her a sustaining "sense of the freshness and the wonder which life in natural surroundings daily brings and a joy in the freedom and beauty and peace that exists in a world apart from human beings." (Reben, The Healing Woods, 1952 p. 250). Her tale of the "Healing Woods" confirms in a lyrical way what many found true before and since.

More famously, perhaps, in 1901, Theodore Roosevelt, then vice president of the United States, was on Mount Marcy in the ADKs, enjoying a hike and views of the forest and lakes below, when he received word that McKinley had been shot. He was rushed by stagecoach and train to Buffalo, New York, and inaugurated as our twenty sixth president. Also, in 1926, President Coolidge made "White Pine Camp" at Paul Smith's in the Adirondacks his summer White House so that he could rest from the stresses of life in Washington, D.C.

Today, New York State itself is heavily populated. Twenty million people live there, 92% of whom live in the New York City Metropolitan area. There are five other major cities in New York State, none of which are in the Adirondacks. Only 130,000 full time residents and 200,000 part timers live in the Adirondacks which comprises 20% of the state's area.

The Adirondack Forest serves as a huge water treatment facility for all those people, gathering rain, filtering it, and aerating it. Precipitation may rest in bogs and swamps, (the nurseries of animal life) and in ponds and lakes. Sooner or later, the water passes through soil, through sand, gravel, and rocks, and is directed onto the larger ponds, lakes, streams, and rivers of the Adirondacks. The ADKs include the headwaters of five major drainage basins: Lake Champlain and the Hudson, Black, St. Lawrence, and Mohawk Rivers. These drainages provide clean water for millions of people.

The Forest also serves us for climate and air quality control. Its vast ecosystem photosynthesizes immense amounts of carbon dioxide; its trees serve as a huge carbon sink, and its fresh oxygen-enriched air is well known for its health benefits.

The area has largely escaped suburban blight to date due to the state legislature's actions over 100 years ago. In 1894, the state adopted the "Forever Wild Clause," severely restricting how the 2.6 million acre Forest Preserve (State owned) lands could be used. Almost 1 million acres were designated "Wilderness" and another 1.6 million acres as protected woodlands and wetlands. In 1912 the legislature clarified that privately held lands (another 2.6 million acres) be included within the "Blue Line" (A blue line drawn on a map in 1891 designated the area to be protected).

The Adirondack Park Agency (APA) was officially created in 1971 to regulate privately held lands. The APA essentially creates and enforces zoning laws that municipalities, developers, businesses, and homeowners are subject to. It remains controversial as it enforces regulations meant to balance economics with the preservation of clean water and air, carbon sequestration, biodiversity, and scenery. The Park as a whole remains the largest undeveloped area east of the Rocky Mountains.

The ADK Forest is one of the largest intact temperate forest ecosystems in the world. Yet only a few patches of old growth forest remain. On the YouTube channel "Adirondack Old Growth Forests- A National Treasure" you can learn only 250,000 acres of the 6 million acre Adirondack Park have never been logged. These acres are comprised of the climax vegetation: sugar maple, beech, and hemlock, and birch, spruce, fir, and larch.

Mature secondary growth has made a significant comeback, as have populations of deer, moose, and beaver. A few other fur-bearers are occasionally spotted in the remotest of areas.

These forests are not untouched though by human activity. Acid rain, noise, and particulate pollution, introduced pathogens such as birch-blight, pests such as gypsy moths, and plants such as milfoil have invaded and put the ecosystem at risk.

We can thank those who have loved the ADK Forest for their actions protecting this majestic, life-supporting ecosystem. The Adirondack Council has worked to clarify what needs to be done to leave it, that is, to "preserve the legacy of the Adirondacks for current and future generations," priorities for 2024 as guided by the VISION 2050 report. ("State of the Park" 2023-2024, p 4).

Recently, Adirondack Forest Bathing has become an accessible way for people in the area needing a brief restorative experience to safely immerse in and meditate on the natural beauty of the Adirondacks while they escape the stresses of modern life.

It is my hope that you have thoroughly enjoyed that endeavor!

PART IV: CITATIONS AND RESOURCES

"Association of Nature and Forest Therapy Guides & Programs | ANFT Forest Therapy."

Www.natureandforesttherapy.earth, www.anft.earth. Accessed 5 July 2024.

Charles Albert Sleicher. *The Adirondacks*. First ed., New York , Exposition Press , 1960.

Chorba, Holly. *A Forest Fungi Bath* . New York, RiverFlow Studio, 2017.

Clement , Josh, and Ed Kanze. "Curiously Adirondack ." *Josh Clement Productions.com* . Accessed 2023.

Clifford, M. Amos. *Your Guide to Forest Bathing : Experience the Healing Power of Nature*. Newburyport, MA, Conari Press, RED WHEEL/WEISER LLC, 2018.

DeSormo, Maitland . *The Heydays of the Adirondacks*. Second Printing ed., P.O. Drawer 209 Saranac Lake, NY 12983, Adirondack Yesteryears Inc. , 1974. Printed in USA by The George Little Press, Burlington, Vt. LCC#: 74-84746

"EDF Impact 2023 - EDF Impact 2023." *EDF Impact 2023*, EDF.org , 16 Nov. 2022, impact2023.edf.org. Accessed 2023. 257 Park Avenue South, New York, NY 10010.

Edmondson, Brad. *A Wild Idea: How the Environmental Movement Tamed the Adirondacks*. Ithaca [New York], Cornell University Press, 2021.

ES11. "State of the Park." *Www.adirondackcouncil.org*, Adirondack Council, 2023, www.adirondackcouncil.org. Accessed 12 Dec. 2023.

"Finding Solutions in Nature." *Global Reach, Local Impact*, no. EDF Impact 2023, 2023, pp. 10–11, impact2023.edf.org. Accessed 2024. 257 Park Avenue South, New York, NY 10010.

Flynn, Andy, and Friends. *New York's Adirondack Park, a User's Guide*. 2013BC. Saranac Lake, NY, Hungry Bear Publishing, 2013, pp. 1–96.

Gibbons, Helene. *Adirondack Riverwalking*, Adirondack Website Design, 5 July 2023, www.AdirondackRiverwalking.com. Accessed 5 July 2024.

Hayes, Arthur. *Lake Placid, Its Early History and Development*. Lake George, NY, Adirondack Resorts Press, Inc., 1946.

Hochschild, Harold K. *Life and Leisure in the Adirondack Backwoods*. 3rd printing ed., Blue Mountain Lake, NY, Adirondack Museum of the Adirondack Historical Association, 1962.

Kaiser, Harvey H. *Great Camps of the Adirondacks*. David R. Godine Publisher, 1 July 2003.

Kanze, Edward. *Adirondack*. SUNY Press, 15 May 2014.

Krempa, Francesca. "A Dose of Nature." *Adirondack Explorer*, vol. 2022 Outings Guide, 2022, pp. 14–16.

Lynch, Mike. "A Healthy Sojourn." *Adirondack Explorer*, no. 2022 Outings Guide, 2022, pp. 10–12.

McMartin, Barbara. *Hides, Hemlocks and Adirondack History.* Utica, NY, North County Books, 1992.

Mitchell, Debra. "A Forest Therapy Walk ." Received by Holly Chorba, 3 2023. an Adirondack Mountain Club Laurentian Chapter event.

Mitchell, Debra . *Forest Therapy Walk.* ADK Mt. Club Forest Therapy Walk. Live Talk.

O'Shea, Peter V. *The Great South Woods.* North Country Books, 1 Oct. 2000.

Reben, Martha. *The Healing Woods* New York, Thomas Y. Crowell Company, 1952. LCC:: 52-7034.

Rubin, Gretchen. *Life in Five Senses.* Crown, 18 Apr. 2023. Accessed 5 July 2024.

Schneider, Paul. *The Adirondacks: A History of America's First Wilderness.* New York, H. Holt and Co, 1998.

Stanton, Kent. "Adirondack Old Growth Forests- a National Treasure." *Youtube.* Accessed 2023.

Sulfoff, Steve. "A Healthy Sojourn (Mike Lynch); A Dose of Nature (Francesca Krempa), Tranquility as Cold River City (Betsy Keeps)". *Adirondack Explorer,* Tracy Ormsbee, 2022, www.adirondackexplorer.org. Accessed 2024. Print editions of the Outings Guide are available each year.

Thoreau, Henry David. *Walden.* London Vintage, 9 Aug. 1854.

Wohlleben, Peter. *HIDDEN LIFE of TREES : What They Feel, How They Communicate?Discoveries from a Secret World.* William Collins, 2018.

Wuerthner, George. *The Adirondacks.* Vol. New York Geographic series, no. 1, Helena, Montana , American Geographic Publishing, 1988.

www.AdirondackWebsiteDesign.com, Adirondack Website Design ~, and Helene Gibbons . "Adirondack Riverwalking and Forest Bathing." *Adirondack Riverwalking and Forest Bathing*, AdirondackRiverwalking & Forest Bathing, LLC and www.AdirondackRiverwalking.com,2023, www.adirondackriverwalking.com. Accessed 29 June 2024.

Six Nations Iroquois Cultural Center, www.6nicc.com . Accessed 5 July 2024. Copyright Six Nations Cultural Center. Design by Rainbow Graphics.

www.ingramcontent.com/pod-product-compliance
Lightning Source LLC
Chambersburg PA
CBHW052033030426
42337CB00027B/4992